W9-BXN-649

HELPING SCHOOLCHILDREN
COPE WITH ANGER

The Guilford School Practitioner Series

EDITORS

STEPHEN N. ELLIOTT, PhD
University of Wisconsin–Madison

JOSEPH C. WITT, PhD
Louisiana State University, Baton Rouge

Recent Volumes

Helping Schoolchildren Cope with Anger

A COGNITIVE-BEHAVIORAL INTERVENTION

◆◆◆

Jim Larson 1942-
John E. Lochman

◆

Foreword by Donald Meichenbaum

THE GUILFORD PRESS
New York   London

© 2002 The Guilford Press
A Division of Guilford Publications, Inc.
72 Spring Street, New York, NY 10012
www.guilford.com

Printed in the United States of America

This book is printed on acid-free paper.

Last digit is print number: 9   8   7   6   5   4   3   2   1

Library of Congress Cataloging-in-Publication Data
Larson, Jim, 1942–
    Helping schoolchildren cope with anger: a cognitive-
  behavioral intervention / Jim Larson, John E. Lochman;
  foreword by Donald Meichenbaum.
       p. cm.—(The Guilford school practitioner series)
    Includes bibliographical references and index.
    ISBN 1-57230-728-5
    1. Aggressiveness in children—Treatment.   2. Cognitive
  therapy for children.   3. Children—Mental health
  services.   4. Oppositional defiant disorder in children—
  Treatment   I. Lochman, John E.   II. Title.   III. Series.

  RJ506.A35 L37 2002
  618.92'89—dc21
                                                  2001056923

About the Authors

◆

Jim Larson, PhD, is Professor of Psychology and Director of the School Psychology Program at the University of Wisconsin–Whitewater. He is also a member of the Scientific Board of the Melissa Institute for Violence Prevention and Treatment of Victims of Violence. Before moving to the University of Wisconsin–Whitewater, Dr. Larson was a school psychologist with the Milwaukee Public Schools in Milwaukee, Wisconsin, and the lead psychologist with the Milwaukee schools' Violence Prevention Program. His principal research interests include the treatment of aggression in children and adolescents, school violence prevention, and training procedures in school psychology.

John E. Lochman, PhD, is Professor and Saxon Chairholder in Clinical Psychology at the University of Alabama. He is also an Adjunct Professor in the Department of Psychiatry and Behavioral Sciences at the Duke University Medical Center. Dr. Lochman's primary research interests include examining the short- and long-term effects of intervention programs provided to high-risk children and adolescents. The school-based and community-based prevention programs he has examined (Anger Coping Program, Coping Power Program, Fast Track Program) use cognitive-behavioral, social problem-solving and social skills training approaches with children, and behavioral training with parents.

Foreword

♦

Seriously aggressive behaviors occur in approximately 5–10% of children, with boys outnumbering girls by almost 3 to 1. The rate of diagnosable conduct disorders has been found to be 6–16% in boys and 2–9% in girls. Such early aggressive behaviors, especially when they occur in combination with poor peer relationships, academic failure, and faulty parenting practices, have proven to be forerunners of later aggressive behavior. The need to develop effective interventions that will avert this developmental trajectory is urgent.

Two leaders in the field, Jim Larson and John Lochman, have brought their clinical perspicacity, school "savvy," and theoretical and empirical expertise together in a timely, well-designed book that will be eagerly welcomed by both school and clinical practitioners. The book focuses on a group intervention that is designed for 8- to 12-year-olds and employs an array of cognitive-behavioral interventions. In a how-to, "nuts-and-bolts" approach, Larson and Lochman describe the various ways group leaders, in collaboration with teachers, school administrators, and parents, can implement effective interventions.

One of the book's primary messages is that "treatment is not only about change, it is about generalization of that change." All too often intervention programs have adopted a "train and hope" approach, but they have failed to build in—from the outset—guidelines for fostering transfer across settings and over time. Larson and Lochman provide a variety of suggestions about how to enhance generalization, including the following:

1. The need to work collaboratively with teachers, administrators, and parents.
2. Use of goal-setting and self-monitoring procedures that participants are required to use across settings.
3. Use of explicit parent training programs.
4. Placing trained students in a consultative mode by having them make training videotapes and by being placed in positions of responsibility, teaching skills to younger children.
5. Having an alumni club of group graduates.
6. Using a primary preventative schoolwide intervention for peers.
7. Providing extended group and individualized training where indicated, so students can develop mastery of anger-control strategies.
8. Training problem-solving metacognitive executive skills and strategies that can be applied across settings.
9. Building in relapse prevention and self-attribution ("taking credit") skills.
10. Providing follow-up booster sessions.
11. Tailoring interventions to the developmental needs of the participants and being sensitive to cultural and gender differences.

The reader will notice that the book embeds these practical guidelines in a heuristically sound theoretical framework of social information processing. As Larson and Lochman observe, research is now under way to further evaluate, in its various forms in other school settings, the intervention that is the central topic of the book. Future versions of the Anger Coping Program will have to take into consideration the increasing recognition of the roles that cognitive and temperament factors (e.g., low cognitive ability, oppositionality, harm avoidance, and callousness) play in the development of antisocial behaviors (see Lahey, Waldman, & McBurnett, 2001). Future intervention programs will likely have to teach significant others how to adapt and influence these temperament factors, as well as teach skills to "high-risk" children. Furthermore, future interventions have to be informed by the research showing that approximately 50 to 60% of children who evidence high levels of conduct disorders in early childhood desist in these disorders in adolescence (Derzon,

2001). A critical question for future research is whether the skills discussed in this book are those used by children who desist. The answer to this question will help fine-tune future generations of the Anger Coping Program.

   In the meanwhile, kudos to Larson and Lochman for an informative, practical, well-designed, and thoughtful book. We are in your debt!

DONALD MEICHENBAUM, PhD
University of Waterloo
The Melissa Institute for Violence
Prevention and Treatment of Victims of Violence
Miami, Florida

Preface

♦

Events over the past few years have brought a sobering realization to the general public that the time has come to re-examine the long-held belief that schools are a "safe haven" for children. Familiar locales like Paducah, Jonesboro, Springfield, and Littleton irrevocably affected the sense of security that so many parents in the United States felt. School-based multiple homicides have challenged the most firmly held beliefs about safety in the classroom.

Yet as horrifying as school shootings may be, a reflective examination of the base rates reassures us of how very rare they truly are. Schools are still the safest places for children to be on a daily basis. In fact, data from the National School Safety Center (2001) confirm that the actual number of single homicides in the school setting has declined 63% over the past decade.

If this is so, why did we choose to write a book about treating aggressive children in the schools? Because whereas *homicide* is on the decline, *interpersonal physical aggression* among students is not. The problem of school violence is not limited to the rare homicide. Data from a combined report by the United States Departments of Education and Justice revealed that approximately 15% of high school students reported that they engaged in a physical fight on school property in the past 30 days (Kaufman et al., 2000). Not all children who are aggressive in the elementary schools go on to become adolescent fighters and victimizers, but early, chronic aggression is enough of a risk factor to warrant being taken very seriously. The collaboration that has resulted in this book is a reflection of our understanding of that seriousness.

The plan for this book resulted from a meeting the two of us held at the National Association of School Psychologists in Chicago in the mid-1990s. Research on the Anger Coping Program had been under way for well over a decade, yet it was clear to us that this potentially important intervention was still the domain of a small circle of researchers and very few practitioners. In our work with school systems, we were aware that most counselors and school psychologists were eager to help address the problem of school violence but were uncertain as to what skills to use to meet the treatment needs of aggressive students. Both of us had done training workshops around the country, but clearly the need went well beyond our limited capacities. We decided to link our Anger Coping Program with our combined experience and scholarship to create a convenient and reliable resource for practitioners.

We have produced what we believe to be a useful, "practitioner-friendly" book about how to intervene effectively with angry, aggressive children. This is a book for school psychologists, counselors, and other helping professionals who work with 8- to 12-year-old children in school or school-like settings. With certain adaptations, mental health professionals in residential or other clinic settings will also find it particularly useful.

Group treatment with aggressive, externalizing children can be a considerable challenge, particularly for those who lack experience. Therapeutic techniques and procedures are rarely addressed comprehensively at the preservice level, so most practitioners are left to acquire the skills on their own. As a result, these children can be left completely unserved or, as is often the case, inadequately served with efforts better designed for less challenging children. The treatment procedures described in this book are empirically based and arise out of both authors' controlled research and years of clinical experience with aggressive children. An effort has been made to combine the extensive body of research with more practical clinical experiential acumen: procedures, hints, and suggestions that have proven themselves useful over the years.

Chapters 1 and 2 provide a solid foundation in the many issues associated with the development of aggression and a guiding theoretical foundation for the Anger Coping Program. These will be particularly useful for readers with little or no training background in aggression or cognitive-behavioral theory and will serve as a helpful refresher for the more experienced practitioner. The careful study of these two chapters is an important prerequisite to the more "hands-on" chapters to follow.

Chapters 3–5 guide the practitioner through the essential, practical steps necessary for an effective intervention. Unlike some other counseling techniques, the Anger Coping Program is a true schoolwide collaboration, with critical roles for the most influential adults, such as teachers, administrators, and parents. The intervention is "multisystemic" in that it encourages a collaboration among the systems of counseling, teaching, and discipline in the effort to effect skills acquisition and generalization. The critical roles of each of these systems and the techniques for their involvement are explained in depth.

Just ahead of the actual treatment manual itself, Chapter 6 reviews the empirical evidence for the effectiveness of the Anger Coping Program. It can be argued that this is the most important chapter. The need for practitioners to understand and utilize empirically based interventions in their work with all children cannot be overstated. Schools in particular are ideal locations for effecting positive therapeutic and behavioral change but only if the efforts to do so are grounded in "what works." The available time with the school day is too short, the personnel costs are too high, and the risks to the children are too great to engage in unsupported "counsel and hope" procedures.

The last section of the book contains the complete, step-by-step treatment manual, along with helpful suggestions, a "Frequently Asked Questions" chapter, and useful appendices. Whereas the manual carefully outlines the empirically supported treatment procedures, it not a "cookie-cutter" approach by any means. Experienced clinicians are encouraged to adjust and supplement the training to meet the specific needs of each group of children while maintaining critical treatment integrity.

In closing, we would like to applaud those practitioners who have chosen the often daunting task of skills training with aggressive children. In most schools, there are populations of children with arguably equivalent needs for mental health services who may present a somewhat lesser challenge in the small group setting. Yet, it is hard to imagine that there are children whose risk for later-life negative outcomes is greater. In these times when schools and the mental health community are under fire to "do something" about violence in society, practitioners who choose to take up the challenge deserve recognition.

JIM LARSON, PhD
JOHN E. LOCHMAN, PhD

Acknowledgments

♦

I wish to express my appreciation to all of my students over the past decade who, through their work with the Anger Coping Program, have helped me to better understand what it means to "do that first group." Thanks also go to Byron and Judith McBride, Donald Meichenbaum, and R. T. Busse for inspiration and assistance, past and present. Special appreciation goes out to school psychologist Wanda Alvarado-Rodriguez for her valuable work on the Spanish translations. Gracias, Wanda! Thanks also to my coauthor, John Lochman, whose dedication to science in the service of children is a model for us all. And, most important, to my parents, to my spouse, Kathy, and my son, Jeremy, I offer my heartfelt thanks for your years of understanding, patience, and undying support in all I do. I am truly blessed by you all.

JIM LARSON

I make acknowledgment here of grants from the National Institute of Mental Health, the National Institute on Drug Abuse, the Center for Substance Abuse Prevention within the Substance Abuse and Mental Health Services Administration, the U.S. Department of Justice, and the Centers for Disease Control and Prevention, all of which have supported the intervention research on the Anger Coping Program and related cognitive-behavioral programs described in this book. I wish to recognize my colleagues, especially Mike Nelson, Louise Lampron, John Curry, John Coie, and Karen Wells, who have collaborated in the development and evaluation of the Anger Coping Program, as well as the graduate students, interns, postdoctoral fellows, school counselors, and school psychologists who, through their experience and feedback in leading Anger Coping groups, have helped to refine the program over the past two decades. I express my deep appreciation to Jim Larson for his vision in planning this book, and for his enthusiasm, persistence, and outstanding commitment to disseminating empirically supported interventions for children. I also wish to thank my wife, Linda, my daughters, Lisa and Kara, and my son, Bryan, for their unfailing support and encouragement of this work over the years.

JOHN E. LOCHMAN

Contents

♦

CHAPTER 1

♦♦♦

The Development of Aggression

♦

SCENE 1

Seven-year-old Robert W took his place in line at the school doorway off the playground, preparing to re-enter the building following recess. He held the classroom's basketball under his arm while he poked his finger at the back of the girl in front of him, hoping to provoke a little rise. Casey R, standing behind Robert, sensed an opportunity for fun and snatched the basketball out of Robert's grasp, giggling loudly. Robert whirled, faced the laughing Casey, and threw himself upon him. Both boys crashed to the pavement, with Casey's head banging hard against the blacktop, opening a bloody gash. Robert straddled the wailing child and pummeled him in the face with both fists until the supervising teacher managed to pull him off.

SCENE 2

Steven C worked the combination lock for his locker, relieved that another day in the sixth grade was finally over and he could head for home. The 15 minutes he'd spent discussing his social studies project after the bell had allowed much of the school to empty, and the third floor hall was uncommonly quiet. Opening the locker door, he reached for his new NBA warm-up jacket and suddenly felt a presence beside him.

He turned and stood face to face with another sixth-grade student, Brian K. Brian was well known among the sixth graders, especially the smaller ones. He was big, intimidating, and mean, and he hung out with a small crowd of equally detestable bullies.

Before Steven could react, Brian's right hand lashed up and gripped him by the neck, knocking his head back against the locker.

"The jacket is just my brother's size. I think I'll take it." He gripped Steven's neck tighter as he pulled the jacket from the locker, a blank, almost calm, look on his face.

"Tell anyone and you're dead meat," he growled, banging Steven's head hard against the locker for emphasis.

Scenes such as these play out in schools around the world. Children and youth aggressing against one another within the school environment has become one of the most significant social concerns of the past decade. Formerly considered "safe havens," schools in some areas of the United States often mirror the violence and danger of their hostile surrounding neighborhoods. Weapon carrying, robberies, and fights are occurring at high levels in U.S. schools (Kingery, Coggeshall, & Alford, 1998). The results of a recent national survey show that more than 8% of students report having been criminally victimized at school, and 12% of all elementary school teachers were threatened with injury by a student (Kaufmann et al., 2000). Little wonder that a recent Phi Delta Kappa/Gallup poll on citizens' concerns ranked lack of discipline, fighting, violence, and gangs as the top problems confronting U.S. schools (Rose & Gallup, 2000).

NEW QUESTIONS FOR SCHOOL PRACTITIONERS

Why do they act that way? How is it that kids from the same community, in the same grade, in the same classroom, can be so different?

Why can some kids take a joke and laugh, whereas other kids get angry and start swinging? Were they born that way or did they learn it somehow? Isn't aggression among young boys normal and won't they outgrow it?

Did the adolescent bully in the preceding vignette give us any hints when he was younger that he might be headed this way by the sixth grade? Is there some sort of a *developmental trajectory* for adolescent aggression? Once started, can this trajectory be altered in a positive direction, or is antisocial behavior ultimately inevitable? Was it simply Brian's "fate" to end up assaulting fellow students?

It has not been typical for school practitioners to ask these questions; this has been more the home turf of developmental, cognitive, and behavioral psychologists who spend their careers—and a staggering amount of private and federal grant money—trying to sort out the answers. Yet although it has not been *typical* in the past for school personnel to investigate the theoretical and developmental psychology of aggression, it has now become *essential*.

In order to intervene effectively in the lives of aggressive children and youth, school personnel must have an understanding of what we currently know about the etiology and development of aggression. Because not all children come to aggressive behavior by the same pathway, developing informed hypotheses about each individual will unquestionably aid in the creation of effective interventions.

Why is aggression among school-age children of such concern? Isn't rough-and-tumble play normal among children, and won't those mean little boys who fight all the time just grow out of it?

Yes, rough-and-tumble play is both normal and common among school-age children, especially boys. Spend any amount of time watching the elementary school recess at virtually any school across the country and be assured.

But, no, the picture for the young fighters is bleak. In fact, there is not a strong likelihood that the children who are demonstrating nonplayful, aggressive behavior at a young age will "just grow out of it." Rather, there is a stronger likelihood that this behavior is a precursor of more violent behaviors to come (Eron, Huesmann, Dubow, Romanoff, & Yarmel, 1987; Loeber, 1990). Indeed, the strongest *single predictor* of an individual's risk of perpetrating violence as an adolescent is a history of having engaged in aggressive behavior as a child (Eron & Slaby, 1994).

HISTORICAL AND CURRENT CONCEPTUALIZATIONS OF AGGRESSION

It might be said that the "modern" era of conceptualizing aggression was ushered in by Dollard, Doob, Miller, Mowrer, and Sears (1939) in their book, *Frustration and Aggression*. These authors held that it was emotional arousal influenced by externally driven events—that is, frustrating experiences or goal blocking—that caused human aggression. All aggression, they theorized, had a goal of injuring another person. This is the essence of what is known as the "hostile aggression" perspective: Injurious intent is an essential aspect. In other words, Dollard et al. (1939) believed that every aggressive act (1) arose out of negative emotionality and (2) was designed to hurt the person or object of the aggression.

This perspective made intuitive sense. Most readers can recall at one time or another having lost their tempers, usually out of frustration directed at another's misbehavior, and then either striking out at that person or wanting to. Although subsequent research has questioned the inevitability of the frustration–aggression link, Pepler and Slaby (1994) observed that the theory "succeeded in shifting attention from explanatory factors that were internal and currently unchangeable to factors that were external and potentially controllable" (p. 28).

Is all aggression, however, merely the result of emotional arousal, such as occurs when an individual is frustrated or angry? Recall the two examples of aggressive students offered at the beginning of this book. In the first example, Robert W was angry at the boy who took his basketball and set upon him aggressively. Clearly, the child was emotionally aroused. The goal of this form of aggression was to inflict harm upon the source of his anger; this action is clearly representative of *hostile aggression.*

However, in the second example, the bully had a grip on Steven's throat and banged his head against the locker with "a blank, almost calm, look on his face." Little or no emotional arousal here, yet plenty of aggression. How is that explained? In this case, the aggressor wasn't angry or frustrated, but he was motivated to acquire something. This is termed *instrumental aggression.* The goal of the bully's behavior was not his victim's pain; it was his victim's jacket. His aggression was not motivated by an internal emotional arousal; it was motivated by the potential for external reward.

Kenneth Dodge (1991) has attempted to offer a unifying theory of aggression in children and youth. Dodge refers to those acts of aggression that are more emotionally driven as *reactive aggression* and those that are more instrumentally driven as *proactive aggression.* This conceptualization can be extremely useful for school personnel, particularly as efforts are put forward for prevention and intervention. Let's look at the two more closely.

Dodge (1991) offered prototypical examples of children who are inclined toward reactive and proactive aggression. He cautioned, however, that these are very rarely pure types, except in extreme cases. "All behaviors have aspects of reaction and proaction, in that one can make guesses regarding the precipitants as well as the functions of all behaviors" (Dodge, 1991, p. 206). Consider Billy, a child who uses proactive aggression:

> The first boy, Billy, is 12 years old and has been arrested four times for vandalism, theft, and similar offenses. He is reported to be a major behavior problem in school. He is a bully among his peers, in that he regularly coerces other boys into deferring to him. He teases peers, threatens them, dominates them, laughs at them, and starts fights with them. (p. 201)

Proactively aggressive children tend to be the bullies in school. Their aggression features relatively little in the way of observable emotion. They may be disliked by their peers, though are often seen to have leadership qualities and an agreeable sense of humor. Their experience is one of positive outcomes for their own aggressive behavior and an abundance of observable violence among family, in the neighborhood, and/or on television. Dodge (1991) also offered the case of Reid, a child inclined to reactive aggression.

> The second boy, Reid, is also 12 years old. He has been arrested for assault on his teacher. One day following her ridicule of him for failing an exam, he pulled a knife on her in the school parking lot and cut her in the arm. He is also considered highly aggressive and socially rejected among peers, but he doesn't seem to start fights so much as he escalates conflicts and can't avoid them. He overreacts to minor provocations and is viewed as volatile and short-tempered. (p. 201)

Reactively aggressive children are the students with hot tempers who seemed to get riled into anger and aggression at the slightest provocation. They often leave school personnel scratching their heads after a blow-up, and asking, "What was *that* all about?" They are almost universally disliked and rejected by peers. They tend to be hypervigilant for aggressive cues in their environment and routinely misinterpret the intentions of peers as hostile.

How do children come to these forms of aggression? Is it biology or something in the child's inborn temperament? Is aggressive behavior learned, and if so, how and where does this learning take place?

THE DEVELOPMENT OF AGGRESSIVE BEHAVIOR

This section briefly discusses three major theoretical positions on the development and maintenance of aggression in children and adolescents: social learning theory, social information processing, and coercive family process. These are not, by any means, the exhaustive positions on the subject. They are, however, theories well supported in the empirical literature and those that seem to have the most heuristic value for school practitioners.

Social Learning Theory

Through much of the last 40 years, Albert Bandura and his colleagues (e.g., Bandura, 1971, 1973, 1983; Bandura & Walters, 1959) have explored the notion that aggressive behaviors are learned and governable, not inborn and uncontrollable. "Aggressive behavior is learned through essentially the same processes as those regulating the acquisition of any other form of behavior" (Bandura, 1973, p. 68). Just because we observe people spending enormous sums of money on fancy television and video gear is no reason to then conclude that such behavior is being impelled by a biologically determined inner drive for television watching. The same reasoning applies to aggressive behavior. Indeed, any highly motivated behavior, whether television watching or punching an obnoxious harasser in the nose, is learned in essentially the same fashion.

This conceptualization of aggression is subsumed under Bandura's *social learning theory*. One can construe social learning theory as "the thinking person's behaviorism." Unlike fellow behaviorists, such as B. F. Skinner, who proposed that all behavior is externally controlled through differential reinforcement and punishment contingencies, Bandura posited that humans are "thinking organisms possessing capabilities that provide [them] with some power of self-direction" (Bandura, 1973, p. 42). In other words, human beings have minds with which to think about their behavior, to imagine new behaviors, to consider the consequences of their behavior, and to draw conclusions by watching others behave. Let us now look at the essential principles of social learning theory and how the theory explains the development of aggressive behavior.

Observational Learning

According to the social learning approach, new behaviors are learned either through experiencing the behavior directly or by observing the behavior of other people. On a daily basis, individuals are confronted with various situations that they must deal with. Sometimes they respond effectively and sometimes they don't. The more effective responses produce favorable results and remain in the behavioral repertoire, whereas the ineffectual ones are discarded (Bandura, 1973). But if we had to experience every type of situation before deciding on an appropriate response, we would progress painfully slowly in adapting to our environment! If we watched a friend walking in front us slip and fall on an icy sidewalk, we wouldn't have to keep walking and slip too before we decided to adjust our gait; we would have learned by *observing* our friend's misfortune.

Children learn aggressive behavior patterns in part by observing the consequences of aggression for others. Children reared in environments where they observe role models for whom aggression usually has positive consequences may learn that aggressive behavior can work for them too. Younger siblings who watch their brothers or sisters regularly get what they want through intimidation, coercion, or direct force—without regular negative outcomes—are more likely to choose similar strategies themselves.

Bandura and colleagues' laboratory work (see Bandura, 1983, for a review) has demonstrated the power of observational learning in regard to the aggressive behavior of young children. In numerous instances, children who viewed a model being rewarded for aggressive behavior were more likely to engage in that behavior themselves than were children who observed the model being punished for his or her aggression. Basic, simple aggressive behaviors like hitting and shoving are physically uncomplicated and require little in the way of practice to enact. A four-year-old preschooler who wants another child's toy and who has observed the efficacy of physical aggression at home is at high risk to enact such behavior him- or herself.

The work of Bandura and others has also demonstrated that aggressive modeling does not have to be live to have an effect on the viewer (e.g., Bandura & Barb, 1973; see Thelen, Fry, Feherenbach, & Frautschi, 1979, for a review). Excessive viewing of violent television by children at risk for aggressive behavior has been demonstrated to have significant effects (see Donnerstein, Slaby, & Eron, 1994, for a review). School personnel must be cognizant of the effects on children who are bombarded daily with both live and media models for aggressive behavior.

Direct Experience

Aggressive behavior can also be learned through the differential reinforcement of engaging in the behavior itself. Children who are reared in environments that offer opportunities for positive outcomes following aggressive behavior may learn to use that behavior in other environments. Children who find that their desires for pleasure or control in a household are met with positive outcomes when they bully smaller children or strike out at adults may learn that such behavior "pays off." Parents who regard aggressive play or aggressive problem solving positively (e.g., Child: "Brother hit me!" Parent: "Well, hit him back!") may be unwittingly contributing to later problems at school and in the community. If such behavior has paid off at home for all their young lives, why would these children believe that it will not have similar results in kindergarten?

Conversely, children who find that their aggressive behavior in the home is met with aversive or negative outcomes—such as parental disapproval, time-outs, or other undesirable consequences—may be less likely to select that behavior in other environments. This is particularly so in households where the child is both taught and reinforced for nonaggressive problem solving.

Self-Regulatory Influences

A central insight in social learning theory is that people have the ability to manage their own behavior by self-monitored consequences as well as or better than through consequences from external sources. "There is no more devastating punishment than self-contempt" (Bandura, 1973, p. 48). This is the power of the mind that social learning theory brings to behaviorism. Praising a child for engaging in a behavior that he or she devalues reduces the effect of the praise. For instance, Lochman, Whidby, and FitzGerald (2000) noted that chronically aggressive boys often place high value on revenge behavior. Now, consider a child such as this who places high value on revenge behavior, whose teacher, following an incident, praises him with "I really like the way you are just forgetting about it." As well-meaning as that praise was meant to be and as powerful as teacher approval may be in other circumstances, the child's self-evaluation that "forgetting about it is bad" will outweigh the teacher's. She may be shocked—and personally affronted—to watch him get up and start punching.

Yet later in the day, the teacher may offer a reinforcer to the same child during a math lesson with the remark "I really like the way you are working hard on these problems" and find that the child's attention to the task actually increases. In this case, the child places value on "working hard," so the external reinforcer is consonant with his self-evaluation.

Most problem solving occurs in thought rather than in action (Bandura, 1973; this insight is expanded on in the section on information processing to follow). It is through the mental representation of possible courses of action that human beings are able to regulate their own behavior. The aforementioned child who enacted revenge upon his classmate first cognitively considered alternative actions (e.g., [1] forget about it or [2] punch him), then evaluated the possible consequences of each course of action, and subsequently executed the favored symbolic solution. In this case, though both behaviors were in his repertoire, the child considered the pain of self-contempt for not getting revenge to be more aversive than the school's consequence for fighting, and selected the aggressive response.

According to social learning theory, humans have the capacity for self-regulation, to select behaviors within their repertoires on the basis of anticipated consequences. The setting—or stimulus condition—has an effect on the behavior choice of the individual, as the calculated consequences differ among environments. A fourth-grade pupil out in the street with his friends who is the recipient of a nonverbal taunt from another child is more likely to select an overtly aggressive response than if he were he aware of the same taunt in church or while shopping with his mother.

Different settings provide cues for the individual about what the likely consequences will be and allow him or her to adjust the response accordingly. Some children for whom the community and/or home environments provide settings that cue positive consequences for aggressive responses have an enormously difficult time making the cognitive switch once they are in the school setting.

Summary

According to a social learning theory model, aggressive behavior is acquired and maintained primarily through (1) observational learning from aggressive models, live or in the media; (2) direct experience of rewarding consequences for aggression; or (3) self-regulatory influences (e.g., applying self-reward or punishment and differential application of cognitive feedback processes). In real life, these influences rarely act singly; instead, they interact with each other in a reciprocal process. Children whose experience has taught them to select aggressive responses at high rates learn to expect others to respond aggressively toward them. This expectation further influences the child to act aggressively. Others respond to the child with counteraggression, thus strengthening the initial expectation.

Consider the hypothetical experience of JR, a third-grade pupil. JR is a middle child in a family of five children, all under the age of 10. His home life is fairly chaotic, with the older children left to babysit while the single parent works two low-paying jobs. Lacking other child management skills, the older children control the younger children down the line through physical aggression and intimidation. The television is on constantly, unmonitored by the absent parent and tuned to the highly violent programming preferred by the dominant older child. The neighborhood is made up of other families like JR's, plus an assortment of unemployed single men. The children are only casually monitored in their play with one another, which ensures frequent fights and a "might makes right" ethos. JR has both *observed* and *directly experienced* positive outcomes for aggression both in his home and in his neighborhood.

One morning in school as the class was lining up for drinks at the water fountain, Terrence W, who was standing in front of JR, backed up and stepped on JR's foot.

"Oops," said Terrence, turning around to face JR with a smile and a shrug. JR's life experience was to expect others to be aggressive toward him, to expect positive outcomes from his own aggression, and to value revenge behaviors over the approval of adults in school. He shoved Terrence, knocking him into another child. Terrence came back toward JR with fists raised in a counterattack, thus confirming for JR that his expectation was accurate and his behavior warranted. The fight was on.

Social learning theory is not the *only* explanation as to how children develop the aggressive behavior patterns we see in school; however, it is an empirically supported and useful conceptualization of the process. As we shall see, numerous other factors inside and outside the child and inside and outside the school building play critical roles with some children.

Social Information Processing

We turn now to a related model that seeks to explain how different aggressive behavior patterns develop. Throughout much of the 1980s and into the 1990s, Kenneth Dodge and colleagues (e.g., Crick & Dodge, 1994; Dodge, 1980, 1986, 1991, 1993a; Dodge & Coie, 1987; Dodge & Frame, 1982) have sought to explain aggressive behavior in children through deficiencies in a social information processing model. Information processing is a cognitive psychology model that uses the empirical method of laboratory experimentation to focus on the verbal learning process, with particular attention to short- and long-term memory. It draws heavily from human engineering in its viewpoint that we humans are information processors and decision makers with limits on how much information we can handle (Goetz, Hall, & Fetsco, 1989).

A sequential framework for competent social information processing in children has been offered by Dodge and others (e.g., Hughes & Hall, 1987). This model identifies six "steps," or cognitive operations, that a child needs to enact for competent social problem solving. The empirical basis for this model is reviewed in the next chapter because of its central role in serving as a foundation for the Anger Coping Program. As a working example of the model, think back to our little friend JR, standing in line at the drinking fountain when the fellow in front of him steps back onto JR's foot.

The *encoding process* (Step 1) occurs when an event happens in proximity to an individual and that person gathers information from his or her sensory systems and perceives the event. There is an enormous amount of information presented in the social environment at any given moment, and central to social competency is the ability to select and attend to the relevant cues (Dodge, 1986). As compared with their normally functioning classmates, aggressive children have a strong tendency to selectively attend to hostile cues at higher rates, to the exclusion of the nonhostile cues. Our little third grader, JR, attended to only the hostile cue of Terrence's foot on his, ignoring a clear cue that it was an accident ("Oops") and the gestures of nonhostility (a shrug and a smile).

After the child has selected the cue to which he or she will attend (i.e., encoded it), the child needs to give meaning to it by mental representation and interpretation (Dodge, 1991). In this *representation and interpretation phase* (Step 2), the child must integrate the cue with his or her memory, looking for an understanding of the meaning of the cue. In JR's incident, he interpreted the encoded cues as being hostile even when no evidence of hostile motivation existed, which indicated a hostile attributional bias. This is what Kendall, Ronan, and Epps (1991) referred to as the "tendency to 'assume the worst' regarding the intention of peers in ambiguous (neither hostile nor benign) situations" (p. 345).

After the child has interpreted the situation to his or her satisfaction, this model hypothesizes that the child engages in a *goal selection process* (Step 3), which indicates the child's desired affective or behavioral outcomes for the social interaction (Crick & Dodge, 1994). In the example involving JR, we could hypothesize that his goal was retaliatory, in response to his biased interpretation of hostile intent. Possible parallel goals of status maintenance ("You can't get away with stepping on *my* toe!") or a felt cultural imperative defense might also be hypothesized.

In the fourth step (*response access or construction*) is seen the child's ability to summon up or generate mental representations of possible responses to the encoded and interpreted cue. For example, a child who has had her desk bumped by another pupil may generate the following response choices if she had encoded and represented the bump as accidental: "I could ignore it. I could ask her to apologize. I could get upset and make her feel bad." JR's limited response search capabilities did not allow him to mentally generate nonaggressive responses to hostility (e.g., assertion, humor, appeal to authority), so he generated the aggressive response.

The fifth step in the social information processing model is the *response decision process*, which asks: "Which of the possible responses shall I choose?" Dodge (1986) offered the analogy of a computer chess game. The computer responds to the human player's moves by accessing its memory and generating countermoves and

evaluating the consequences of each move. The size and sophistica-
tion of the computer's memory will allow it to determine the probable
consequences for one, two, three, or more moves ahead. The more
complex the memory and sophisticated the operating system, the
more competent the selected move will be. Our young friend, JR,
evaluated the probable consequences of shoving Terrence for stepping
on his foot as positive and judged that his skills to carry out the response were up to the task. Why didn't he consider any alternative solutions? Didn't he know he would get in trouble for that behavior? Is
it that he doesn't care?

In the *behavioral enactment process* (Step 6), once the child has
selected a response that he or she believes to be optimal, the child proceeds to act it out (Dodge, 1986). To be successful, the child has to
have the necessary behavioral skills in his or her repertoire. For instance, a child may decide that questioning a peer's behavior is the optimal response, but if he or she does not have the verbal skills to carry
it out, the enactment will not be competent (Pepler, King, & Byrd,
1991). Failure to competently enact a selected behavior creates a new
cue and a loop back through the process. Because aggressive children
tend to lack many of the social skills necessary to engage prosocial
problem-resolution strategies, their occasional attempts are incompe-
tently enacted. If JR had selected a nonaggressive response to Terrence, such as asking him to be careful, he would have needed the verbal skills to do it—and to do so without making it sound like a threat.
Such skills involve, among others, word selection, voice tone, facial
expression, and body posture. Although many students learn these social skills easily through home and school modeling and practice, others, like JR, aren't so fortunate.

Coercive Family Process

Lonnie K is 6 years old and in the first grade. He lives with both
parents, a paternal grandfather, one younger and one older
brother. They all reside in the grandfather's home a few blocks
from the school. Lonnie's father is currently unemployed and is
on court probation for assault and criminal damage to property
following an incident at a local tavern. Lonnie's mother is a hair-
dresser at a neighborhood shop. She was recently let go from an
assistant manager position in a nearby town because of absences
she blames on bouts of depression. Lonnie's oldest brother, Ray-

mond, is in the seventh grade in a special education program for emotionally disturbed/behaviorally disordered students and has had a number of contacts with the juvenile court. There have been six calls to Social Services by neighbors over the past 10 years, primarily for suspected neglect of the children.

In his first-grade class, Lonnie presents an enormous behavior problem. He is extremely oppositional to his teacher's requests for compliance, is aggressive toward the other children, and is unable to participate regularly in group games without hitting or pushing another child. He has to be closely monitored on the playground because of his tendency to push children off swings and playground equipment rather than wait his turn. At his best, he can be charming and funny. His teacher laments, however, that "he is growing up to be the same mean kid his older brother is."

In this section, referring to the family of 6-year-old Lonnie K as an example, we investigate the contributions of the home context to the development of aggressive behavior patterns in children. The great body of research in this area has come from Gerald Patterson and his colleagues at the Oregon Social Learning Center (e.g., Patterson, 1982; Patterson, DeBaryshe, & Ramsey, 1989; Patterson, Reid, & Dishion, 1992; Patterson, Reid, Jones, & Conger, 1975; Reid & Patterson, 1991). It was Patterson (1982) who coined the term *coercive family process* to describe a family pattern composed of the interaction between ineffective parent management skills and escalating child behavior problems. This is a family process that actually *trains* children to be aggressive and noncompliant (Patterson, 1982; Patterson et al., 1989).

Lonnie's family demographics include some of the risk factors found to be implicated in the development of aggression in the family context. Low socioeconomic status, substance abuse by parent(s), criminality of parent(s), and maternal depression have all been associated with exacerbating the coercive family process (Kazdin, 1987b; Reid & Patterson, 1991). These demographic factors, singly or together, do not cause aggressive or antisocial behavior to develop, but they do function as significant stressors that can undermine attempts at effective parenting.

It's 7:00 P.M. and Lonnie and his mother are watching a television show, when 12-year-old brother Ray comes in and demands that he be allowed to watch his video. Lonnie stands and complains loudly, only to receive a shove from Ray, who then moves to insert his video in the VCR.

"Tell him I was here first," Lonnie demands of his mother.

"Ray," their mother finally says, looking up from her crossword puzzle. "Lonnie was watching that."

"Tough shit," returns Ray, now easily fending off wild punches thrown by Lonnie. One lands too near his genitals, and Ray boxes Lonnie on the side of his head hard. Lonnie howls in pain and screams at his mother.

"He hit me in the face!"

"Well, you were hitting him," returns his mother. "What did you expect? Now, if you both don't stop hitting, I'll get your father down here."

Lonnie ignores her and begins once again to flail away at his brother. Ray has finally had enough and wraps his arms around Lonnie's neck, squeezing.

When he finally loosens his hold, Lonnie runs from the room, shouting out his new mission to destroy some of Ray's property.

"I'll kill you if you touch my stuff!" shouts Ray, settling down in front of the set.

Their mother shakes her head and returns to her crossword.

This interaction demonstrates two central characteristics of the coercive family process: ineffective parental management of aggressive, noncompliant behavior and the reinforcement of coercive child behaviors. This model posits that the effectiveness with which parents manage the aggressive and noncompliant behaviors of their children plays a critical role in the course of those behaviors as the child grows. In the coercive family, as the children's aggressive behaviors grow more and more frequent and increasingly intense, the parents' attempts to manage them become increasingly inadequate (Reid & Patterson, 1991).

In the preceding example, rather than stepping in to manage the conflict, Lonnie's mother merely sits there making "parental noises." It is not uncommon to find parents, mothers especially, for whom years of ineffective parenting have led to an emotional detachment, often depression. Her vague threat about calling the father down, possibly to engage in physical aggression against the children, is ignored. Lonnie and his brother have presumably learned that she cannot physically control them herself and that her threats are rarely carried out. Consequently, they now control her to a large degree. In addition, the two boys have learned that coercive behavior patterns pay off: Ray knows that he can muscle his way into the television show Lonnie and his mother are watching, without serious opposition. The fact that his mother ultimately allows him to be successful only makes it more likely that he will repeat the behavior in other circumstances.

Patterson and his colleagues found that in families such as this, the effect of inept parenting practices is to permit literally dozens of daily interactions within the family in which coercive child behaviors are directly reinforced (Patterson et al., 1989). At times reinforcement comes through some form of positive regard of the parent for the coercive behavior, such as when a parent laughs at a scene of sibling bullying behavior. In addition, as in the example, instances in which the parent passively allows the child's coercive behavior to be successful (i.e., reinforced) increase the likelihood of later repetition.

The researchers found, however, that most of the reinforcement arises from escape contingencies, or what has been called an attack, counterattack, positive outcome sequence. In such a sequence, when a parent intrudes with a request for compliance (e.g., *attack*: "Go to bed now"), the child learns to use aversive behaviors to escape (*counterattack*: "I ain't going and you can't make me!"). The inept parent, believing that escaping from this aversive interaction with the child is most important, submits (*positive outcome*: "Fine, stay up and be tired all day in school. I don't care"). As an unfortunate consequence, both the child's noncompliant, coercive response and the parent's escape behavior have been reinforced. The stage is set for the sequence to be repeated.

One of the features of the coercive family process is an escalation of the intensity of the coercive interactions (Patterson et al., 1989). Threats become violence, and violence becomes greater violence. With each successive interaction, the potential for either the "attack" or the "counterattack" to escalate in intensity is very real. Among family members, fear of the intensity of the interaction produces children who can control their parents and parents unwilling to discipline their children effectively.

It is nearly 3:30 P.M. and Lonnie is returning from school. He walks through the front door of his home and into the living room. His father is in front of the TV, beer cans spread about. Lonnie is just about to begin a loud complaining script, which has successfully driven his father from the television in the past, when the man stands up from his chair. Lonnie recognizes the hostile, intoxicated look and starts to back away, but not quickly enough. His father grabs him by the front of his shirt and slaps his open palm hard against the side of Lonnie's face.

"Fighting again at school? Got your damn principal callin' me at home? I'll give you all the fighting you want!" his father yells, slamming his hand once again into the struggling boy. The beating continues until Lonnie is finally able to wrest himself free and bolt out the door.

Harsh, inconsistent, physical discipline is often characteristic of the coercive family process (Patterson, 1982). Ineffective parents tend to have a very narrow repertoire of discipline strategies—often limited to either verbal or physical aggression. In addition, when parental discipline is tied too closely to the parent's mood or whim, the outcome is that a certain behavior is ignored one day and punished the next. Parents who ignore (or even encourage) sibling fighting at home, then beat the child for the same behavior in school, are doing more to increase the child's aggression than to eliminate it. Aggressive behavior that is punished with counteraggression and in an unpredictable, erratic fashion becomes extremely resistant to change (Park & Slaby, 1983).

Linkages from coercive family processes to the development of deviant social information processing patterns have been noted. Dodge, Bates, and Pettit (1990) found that children who experienced physical maltreatment when they angered their parents were more likely to direct aggression toward peers who irritate them. The same children displayed more deviant processing styles, that is, they were less attentive to relevant cues, displayed hostile attributional biases, and showed poor solution generating skills (Dodge et al., 1990; Pettit, 1997). It should come as little surprise to find that Lonnie, the youngster in the preceding coercive family example, displayed many of the information-processing deficiencies common to aggressive children.

SUMMARY

As school practitioners consider intervention efforts, a knowledge of the factors involved in the onset and maintenance of chronic aggressive behavior is essential. Social learning theory provides a solid and useful cognitive-behavioral framework upon which to conceptualize the direction of treatment options. The practitioner with this knowledge understands the strength of both observational models and direct experience. Confining all the naughty and aggressive children to a single "behavior disorders" classroom, where they have only negative models, or failing to effectively reinforce prosocial problem solving runs counter to these principles.

The social information processing research of Dodge and others allows the practitioner to hypothesize the existence of both cognitive and behavioral deficits that may be responsive to treatment. Each "step" offers an opportunity for intervention. Through problem solving skills training (e.g., Hughes & Clavell, 1995; Lochman, Lampron, Gemmer, & Harris, 1987), children may be helped to attend to the proper environmental cues, learn to reduce tendencies toward hostile attributional bias, and increase their repertoire of nonaggressive problem-solving strategies.

The research findings of Gerald Patterson and others have demonstrated how family demographics (especially low socioeconomic status), parental characteristics such as criminality and substance abuse, coercive parent–child interactions, and ineffective parental discipline practices can all potentiate one another to create a training environment for aggressive, antisocial behavior in children. Parent management-training procedures offer the practitioner an intervention with considerable promise for treating the antisocial behavior of the child (Kazdin, 1987a, 1995; Larson, 1994). These procedures seek to enhance such parenting skills as nonphysical discipline strategies, child monitoring, and issuing effective compliance directives.

In the next chapter, we review the empirical basis for our model of the emotional and social-cognitive difficulties of aggressive children.

CHAPTER 2

◆◆◆

The Empirical Foundation for a Developmental Model of Aggressive Children's Social-Cognitive and Emotional Difficulties

◆

The occurrence of aggressive and oppositional behaviors is relatively common in mild to moderate forms during the early childhood years. However, most children develop methods for regulating their emotions and impulsive behavior during the elementary school years. Aggressive behavior becomes more clinically significant if the behaviors are highly intense and violent, if they generate significant harm, and if they occur with high frequency (Lochman, 2000c). Seriously aggressive behavior occurs in approximately 5 to 10% of children, and boys with antisocial behavior outnumber girls by two or three to one (Kazdin, 1998; Lochman & Szczepanski, 1999). Rates of conduct disorder are estimated to be in the range of 6 to 16% for boys and 2 to 9% for girls (American Psychiatric Association, 1994). Children are more at risk for continued aggressive and antisocial behavior if they display aggressive behavior in multiple settings (e.g., home, school, and neighborhood) and if they develop "versatile" forms of antisocial behavior, including both overt (assaults, direct threats) and covert (theft) behaviors by early to midadolescence (Lochman, White, Curry & Rumer, 1992; Loeber & Schmalling, 1985).

Loeber (1990) hypothesized that aggressive behavior in elementary school years is part of a developmental trajectory that can lead to adolescent delinquency and conduct disorder. Longitudinal research has documented this evolution of behavioral problems by noting that aggressive behavior and rejection by a child's peers can be additive risk markers for subsequent maladjusted behavior in the middle school years (Coie, Lochman, Terry & Hyman, 1992) and that aggressive behavior is a risk marker for early substance abuse, overt delinquency, and police arrests in the later adolescent years (Coie, Terry, Zakriski, & Lochman, 1995; Lochman & Wayland, 1994).

AGGRESSION AND ANGER

Aggressive behavior in children and adults has been conceptualized as being in part due to an inability to regulate emotional responses to anger-producing stimuli (Lochman, Dunn, & Wagner, 1997). Children's aggressive behavior has been related to intense emotional arousal in general (e.g., Cummings, Iannotti, & Zahn-Waxler, 1985) and to high levels of anger in particular (Eisenberg, Fabes, Nyman, Bernzweig, & Pinuelas, 1994).

When individuals perceive themselves as endangered or threatened, they have common physiological responses at two levels (Goleman, 1995) and can have two types of anger (Lochman et al., 1997). When threat is perceived, the thalamus signals the neocortex, which then processes the perceived causes and possible responses to the threat. The result can be a deliberate, calculated anger response. The action of the amygdala on the adrenocortical branch of the nervous system can create a general background state of action readiness, which can last for hours or for days. This activation can be stimulated by stress of all kinds, and individuals become more prone to serious anger arousal if they are already activated by mild to moderate irritation and frustration. When a person is in this state of readiness, even minor triggers can produce highly intense anger responses. Thus, anger can build on anger (Goleman, 1995). Escalating anger can be the result of a series of perceived provocations, each of which triggers further arousal, which dissipates slowly.

In addition to this first physiological response to perceived threat, the thalamus can also signal the amygdala, and, separate from the collateral cortical processing, the amygdala can directly trigger a surge in heart rate and blood pressure and produce a rage response. This limbic surge can release catecholamines and lead to an energy rush, which may last for a period of only a few minutes. Anger can develop very rapidly because of the initial limbic surge and can be manifest overtly in increased cardiovascular activity. Highly aggressive boys have been found to have lower resting heart rates than nonaggressive boys, but they can display a sharp surge in heart rate following interpersonal provocation (Craven, 1996).

SOCIAL-COGNITIVE MODELS

Angry aggression can be readily conceptualized within a social information-processing model of anger arousal (Crick & Dodge, 1994; Lochman et al., 2000). Many of the most recent interventions for disruptive behavior disorder are based on cognitive-behavioral theories of antisocial and delinquent behavior. The premise behind many of these interventions is that cognitions or thoughts influence the behavior that an individual displays in various situations, and thus alters both the individual's general response (behavioral) patterns and the cognitions that accompany or precede the behaviors. Cognitive-behavioral interventions with aggressive children are thus designed to impact on social behavior and related cognitive and emotional processes. These forms of intervention are based on a social-cognitive theoretical model, which describes social behavior as a function of children's perceptions of their immediate social environment and of their ideas about how to resolve the perceived social conflicts.

Anger Arousal Model

An early form (the Anger Control Program) of our current cognitive-behavioral intervention program was based on an anger arousal model (Lochman, Nelson & Sims, 1981). This model was primarily derived from Novaco's (1978) work with aggressive adults. In this conceptualization of anger arousal, which stressed sequential cognitive processing, the child responded to problems such as interpersonal conflicts or frustrations with environmental obstacles (i.e., difficult schoolwork). However, it was not the stimulus event itself that provoked the child's response, but rather the child's cognitive processing of and about that event. This first stage of cognitive processing was similar to Lazarus's (Smith & Lazarus, 1990) primary appraisal stage and consisted of labeling, attributions, and perceptions of the problem event. The second state of processing, similar to Lazarus's (Smith & Lazarus, 1990) secondary appraisal, consisted of the child's cognitive plan for his or her response to the perceived threat or provocation. This level of cognitive processing was accompanied by anger-related physiological arousal. The anger arousal model indicated that the child's cognitive processing of the problem event and of his or her planned response led to the child's actual behavioral response (ranging from aggression to assertion, passive acceptance, or withdrawal) and to the positive or negative consequences that the child experienced as a result.

The anger arousal model served as the basis for the social-cognitive model in our revised Anger Coping Program (Lochman et al., 1987; Lochman, White & Wayland, 1991; Lochman, FitzGerald, & Whidby, 1999; Lochman et al., 2000). This social-cognitive model stressed the reciprocal interactive relationships between the initial cognitive appraisal of the problem situation, the cognitive appraisal of the problem solutions, the child's physiological arousal, and the behavioral response. The Anger Coping Program introduced the role that labeling emotions, thought processes, and schematic propositions can have in the child's social-cognitive processes. In this model, there is emphasis on the interrelatedness of the different elements of the model, in that all processing steps/components have some influence on all other elements. There is also emphasis on the ongoing nature of interpersonal interaction, as children's responses to various social stimuli lead to sets of new social stimuli to be encountered in the future. The level of physiological arousal will depend on the individual's biological predisposition to become aroused and will vary according to the interpretation of the event. The level of arousal further influences the social problem solving, operating either to intensify the fight-or-flight response or to interfere with the generation of solutions. This model helps to explain the chronic nature of aggressive children's difficulties, as there is emphasis on the ongoing and reciprocal nature of interactions. Thus, aggressive children's difficulties may form a circular pattern, and it may be difficult for them to extricate themselves from the aggressive behavior patterns.

Social Information-Processing Model

As noted in Chapter 1, the social information-processing model developed by Dodge (1993b; Crick & Dodge, 1994; Dodge, Pettit,

McClaskey, & Brown, 1986) explicitly expands on substeps in the child's cognitive processing of social problems and serves as an important heuristic for research with aggressive children. In this model, there are six sequential steps involved in the processing of social information: encoding relevant social cues, interpreting these cues, identifying social goals, generating possible solutions to the perceived problem, evaluating these solutions, and enacting the chosen response. The first two steps involve cognitive processing of the problem event, and Steps 4 and 5 involve cognitive processing about responses. Aggressive children have been found to have difficulties at each of these stages. They are prone to cognitive distortions when encoding incoming social information (Step 1) and when interpreting social events and others' intentions (Step 2). They also appear to have systematic differences in their social goals (Step 3), cognitive deficiencies in generating alternative adaptive solutions for perceived problems (Step 4) and evaluating the consequences for different solutions (Step 5), and behavioral deficiencies in enacting the solution believed to be most appropriate (Step 6) (Lochman et al., 2000).

Considerable research has indicated that aggressive children do exhibit the distortions and deficiencies suggested here. In terms of the initial stage, the encoding of information, aggressive children have been found to recall fewer relevant cues about events (Lochman & Dodge, 1994), to base interpretations of events on fewer cues (Dodge & Newman, 1981; Dodge et al., 1986), to selectively recall and attend to hostile rather than neutral cues (Gouze, 1987; Milich & Dodge, 1984), and to recall the most recent cues in a sequence, with selective inattention to earlier presented cues (Milich & Dodge, 1984). McKinnon, Lamb, Belsky, & Baum (1990) have suggested that these biases at the encoding phase, which involve selective attention to particular cues in the environment, are a direct result of prior social interactions and are, in fact, a logical outcome of the aggressive child's early affectively toned attachment relationships. Accordingly, the child learns to pay attention to interaction patterns and social cues that are emotionally similar to cues he or she has previously experienced; for instance, if a child has experienced primarily negative or aggressive interactions with a parent, he or she will more likely attend to, and process, aggressively toned cues.

At the next stage, interpretation, aggressive children have been shown to have a hostile attributional bias, as they tend to excessively infer that others are acting toward them in a provocative and hostile manner (Dodge et al., 1986; Katsurada & Sugawara, 1998). This attributional bias can be evident in live interactions as well as in hypothetical vignettes (Steinberg & Dodge, 1983), and both aggressive girls (Feldman & Dodge, 1987) and aggressive boys (Guerra & Slaby, 1989; Lochman & Dodge, 1994; Sancilio, Plumert, & Hartup, 1989; Waas, 1988) have been found to have this attributional bias. In addition, in studies of boys' interpersonal perceptions after actual dyadic interactions, Lochman (1987; Lochman & Dodge, 1998) found that aggressive boys have underperceptions of their own aggressive behavior (see themselves as less aggressive than they really are), as well as distorted overperceptions of others' aggression (see others as more aggressive than they are). As a result, aggressive boys develop attributions that assign responsibility for conflict to their peers, rather than assuming responsibility themselves.

The fourth information-processing stage involves a generative process whereby potential solutions for coping with a perceived problem are recalled from memory. At this stage, aggressive children demonstrate deficiencies in both the quality and the quantity of their problem-solving solutions (Lochman, Meyer, Rabiner, & White, 1991). These differences are most pronounced in the quality of the solutions offered. For instance, in response to hypothetical conflicts describing interpersonal conflicts, aggressive children offer fewer verbal assertion solutions (Asarnow & Callan, 1985; Joffe, Dobson, Fine, Marriage, & Haley, 1990; Lochman & Lampron, 1986), fewer compromise solutions (Lochman & Dodge, 1994), more direct action solutions (Lochman & Lampron, 1986), a greater number of help-seeking or adult intervention responses (Asher & Renshaw, 1981; Dodge, Murphy, & Buschbaum, 1984; Lochman, Lampron, & Rabiner, 1989; Rabiner, Lenhart, & Lochman, 1990), and more physically aggressive responses (Pepler, Craig, & Roberts, 1998; Slaby & Guerra, 1988; Waas, 1988; Waas & French, 1989). In terms of the quantity of solutions, there is little evidence that aggressive children overall offer a fewer number of responses (Bloomquist et al., 1997; Rubin, Bream, & Rose-Krasnor, 1991). However, the most severely aggressive and violent youth do have a deficiency in the number of solutions they can generate to resolve social problems (Lochman & Dodge, 1994). The nature of the social problem-solving deficits for aggressive children can vary, depending on their diagnostic classification. Boys with conduct disorder diagnoses produce more aggressive/antisocial solutions in vignettes about conflicts with parents and teachers, and fewer verbal/nonaggressive solutions in peer conflicts, in comparison with boys with oppositional defiant disorder (Dunn, Lochman, & Colder, 1997). Thus, children with conduct disorder have broader problem-solving deficits in multiple interpersonal contexts, in comparison with children with oppositional defiant disorder.

The fifth processing step involves a two-step process: first, identifying the consequences for each of the solutions generated, and second, evaluating each solution and consequence in terms of the individual's desired outcome. In general, aggressive children evaluate aggressive behavior as less negative (Deluty, 1983) and more positive (Crick & Werner, 1998) than children without aggressive behavior difficulties. Children's beliefs about the utility of aggression and about their ability to successfully enact aggressive responses can increase the likelihood of aggression being displayed, as children who hold these beliefs will be more likely to also believe that this type of behavior will help them to achieve their desired goals, which then influences their response decisions (Lochman & Dodge, 1994; Perry, Perry, & Rasmussen, 1986). Recent research has found that these beliefs about the acceptability of aggressive behavior lead to deviant processing of social cues, which in turn lead to children's aggressive behavior (Zelli, Dodge, Lochman, Laird, & the Conduct Problems Prevention Research Group, 1999), indicating that these information-processing steps have reciprocal effects on each other, rather than strictly linear ones.

The final processing stage listed by Dodge et al. (1986) involves behavioral enactment, or displaying the response that was chosen in the previous steps. Aggressive children have been found to be less adept at enacting positive or prosocial interpersonal behaviors (Dodge, et al., 1986). Improving aggressive children's ability to successfully and effectively enact positive behaviors may enhance their beliefs about their ability to engage in these more prosocial behaviors and thus make them more likely to choose such prosocial solutions.

The Crick and Dodge Reformulated Model

Crick and Dodge's (1994) more recent modification of the original model describes more of the on-line processing that actually occurs when individuals are engaged in social interactions. This model also contains an explicit reference to the idea that the consequences of one's behavior will feed back into the system and function as the stimulus for the next interaction. In addition, a new step (the third step) was included in the information-processing model. This step involves a clarification of goals that the individual wishes to attain and involves selecting the desired goal from different possible goals (e.g., to avoid punishment, to get even with another individual, to affiliate). It also involves determining which goal predominates during the particular interaction. The goal that the individual chooses to pursue will then affect the responses generated for resolving the conflict, which occurs in the next processing stage. The children's social goals can be conceptualized as being a part of their stable schemas of interpersonal situations, as discussed in a subsequent section. More generally, schemas (or the database) can be accessed at any of the processing stages and can be influenced by stored knowledge derived from experience in a similar situation. Furthermore, each stage will provide information relevant to the ongoing evolution of schemas, which will then have an impact on future interactions.

Social Information Processing among Subtypes of Aggressive Children

Research has begun to examine whether subtypes of children with specific types of aggressive behavior patterns have different patterns of social-cognitive deficiencies. Dodge and Coie (1987) differentiated between proactive aggressive children, who engage in aggressive behavior in a relatively planned, nonemotional way, and reactive aggressive children, who become impulsively aggressive when they are aroused to anger following perceived provocations. Reactive aggressive children have been found to be more likely to have social-cognitive difficulties throughout the full array of information-processing steps. In particular, they are oversensitive to hostile cues and have higher rates of hostile attributional biases. Proactive aggressive children have been primarily characterized by their relatively high expectations that aggressive behavior will work for them (Dodge, Lochman, Harnish, Bates, & Pettit, 1997). Harsh parenting and neighborhood violence appear to be important factors contributing to the development of reactive aggression and to reactive aggressive children's hostile attributional biases (Lochman & Wells, 1999c; Lochman, Wells, & Colder,

1999). When severely aggressive children and adolescents have been compared with moderately aggressive children, the severely aggressive youth are similarly more likely to display the full array of distortions and deficiencies in their social information processing, and moderately aggressive youth are primarily characterized by having higher expectations that aggression will work and successfully resolve the problem at hand (Lochman & Dodge, 1994). These findings suggest that interventionists should be sensitive to variations in the intensity and topography of children's aggressive behavior, and that these differences will likely require changes in which certain portions of an intervention will be emphasized more for some children than for others.

Role of Schemas in Social Information Processing

Although the reviewed research evidence indicates that aggressive children do have certain difficulties in how they process social information, the variations across subtypes of aggressive children suggest that other cognitive and emotional factors within the children contribute to these processing difficulties (Lochman, Magee, & Pardini, in press). Recent revisions of social-cognitive models have more explicitly examined the role that children's cognitive schemas play in their information processing (Crick & Dodge, 1994; Lochman et al., 2000; Lochman, Wayland, & White, 1993; Lochman, White, & Wayland, 1991). Schemas account for how individuals actively construct their perceptions and experiences, rather than merely being passive receivers and processors of social information (Ingram & Kendall, 1986). Schemas have been defined in somewhat different ways by various theoreticians and researchers, but are commonly regarded as consistent core beliefs and patterns of thinking (Lochman & Lenhart, 1995). These underlying cognitive structures form the basis for individuals' specific perceptions of current events (DeRubeis, Tang, & Beck, 2001). Similar to Adler's concept of "style of life" (Freeman & Leaf, 1989), schemas are cognitive blueprints or master plans that construe, organize, and transform peoples' interpretations and predictions about events in their lives (Kelly, 1955; Mischel, 1990).

Schemas have certain basic attributes (Lochman et al., in press). First, a distinction can be made between *active* schemas, which are often conscious and govern everyday behavior, and *dormant* schemas, of which an individual is typically unaware and emerge only when the individual is faced with specific events or stressors (Lochman & Lenhart, 1995). Dormant schemas are in a state of "chronic accessibility" (Higgins, King, & Marvin, 1982; Mischel, 1990) or state of potential activation, ready to be primed by minimal cues. Thus, an individual's beliefs and expectations, which emerge when the individual is intensely stressed or aroused, may not be at all apparent when the individual is calm and nonaroused.

Second, existing schemas can be either compelling or noncompelling (Freeman & Leaf, 1989). Noncompelling schemas are not strongly held by a person and can be given up easily. In contrast, compelling schemas are strongly entrenched in the person's way of thinking. They promote more filtering and potential distortions of the person's perceptions of self and others (Fiske & Taylor, 1984). Compelling schemas lead individuals to make more rapid judgments about the presence of schema-related traits in self and others, and they often operate outside conscious awareness (Erdley, 1990).

Third, schemas can be more or less permeable. Permeable schemas permit a person to alter his or her interpretation of events through successive approximations, a process identified by Kelly as "constructive alternativism" (1955). A person with relatively permeable schemas can readily adapt his or her schemas to the specific situations and conditions that person encounters, thereby adding new elements and complexity to the schemas. Schemas are typically more permeable and situational as individuals develop and have experiences in a number of situations (Mischel, 1990; Rotter, Chance, & Phares, 1972). Relatively nonpermeable schemas are preemptive, promote rigid black-and-white thinking (Kelly, 1955), and are likely to create rigid expectations that are not open to change based on new information. The process of altering schemas is essentially conservative (Lochman & Dodge,1998), as preexisting beliefs are accepted over new ones, and self-centered, because a person's own personal preexisting beliefs are held more strongly than new information provided by others (Fiske & Taylor, 1984). Nonpermeable schemas are self-maintaining because they lead the individual to seek and recall information that is consistent with his or her conceptions others and self.

Fourth, schemas permit individuals to predict the outcomes of events (Adler, 1964). Schemas allow people to operate efficiently in their social worlds by providing expectations of how others will react and how they will be able to meet their own goals and needs (Lochman & Dodge, 1998).

Schemas within the Social-Cognitive Model

Schemas have been proposed to have a significant impact on the information-processing steps within the social cognition models underlying cognitive-behavioral interventions with aggressive children (Lochman, White, & Wayland, 1991; Lochman et al., 2000). Ingram and Kendall (1986; Kendall, 2000) have organized individuals' cognitive processing of events into four categories in their cognitive taxonomic system. *Cognitive products* are the actual cognitions that individuals have in the present when dealing with events (e.g., attributions, decisions, beliefs, thoughts, recognition of stimuli), and *cognitive operations* are the procedures that process information (e.g., attention, encoding, retrieval). Cognitive operations operate on the immediate stimuli and on schemas to produce cognitive products. Schemas have two forms within the cognitive taxonomic system: cognitive structures and cognitive propositions. *Cognitive structures* are the architecture of the cognitions in memory, the structures by which information is organized and stored. These functional psychological mechanisms store information in both short- and long-term memory, placing information in interconnecting categories and nodes. *Cognitive propositions* form the content within the cognitive structures, and constitute the information that is actually stored. Cognitive propositions include information both in semantic memory (general knowledge that has been acquired and learned) and in episodic memory (personal information gleaned through the person's experiences in the world). In the social-cognitive model, social-cognitive products include elements within the social information-processing steps such as encoded cues, attributions, problem solutions, goals, and anticipated consequences that individuals experience during moment-to-moment processing.

Schematic propositions are those beliefs, ideas, and expectations that can have direct and indirect effects on the social-cognitive products. Schematic propositions include information stored in memory about an individual's beliefs, general social goals, generalized expectations, and understanding of competence and self-worth (Lochman & Lenhart, 1995; Lochman et al., in press).

Direct Effects of Schemas on Social Information Processing

Schemas can influence the sequential steps of information-processing in different ways. Early in the information-processing sequence, when the individual is perceiving and interpreting new social cues, schemas can have a clear direct effect by narrowing the child's attention to certain aspects of the social cue array (e.g., Lochman et al., 1981). A child who believes it is essential to be in control of others and who expects others to try to dominate him or her, often in aversive ways, will attend particularly to verbal and nonverbal signals about someone else's control efforts, easily missing any accompanying signs of the other person's friendliness or attempts to negotiate. Children's schema about control and aggression will also heavily influence the second stage of processing, as the child interprets malevolent meaning and intentions in others' behavior (Lochman et al., in press).

Schemas can also play a significant role in the fifth stage of information processing, as the child anticipates consequences for different problem solutions available to him or her and decides which strategy will be enacted. Social goals (accessed at the third stage of information processing) and outcome expectations are schemas that, from a social learning theory view (Mischel, 1990; Rotter et al., 1972), combine to produce children's potential for behaving in specific ways. When the child places a higher value on certain goals or reinforcements, the child will then engage in behaviors that he or she expects will have a high probability of meeting such goals. Aggressive adolescent boys have been found to place higher value on the social goals of dominance and revenge, and lower value on the social goal of affiliation, than do nonaggressive boys (Lochman, Wayland, & White, 1993). In addition, within the aggressive group, very small differences have been found in the values that aggressive boys assign to dominance, revenge, avoidance, and affiliation goals, indicating that aggressive youth are likely to have a "muddy," or conflicted, goal structure. In one study, there was also a clear relation between social goal choice and problem-solving ability, indicating a direct effect of cognitive schemas on information processing. Aggressive boys proposed fewer bargaining solutions and more aggressive and verbal assertion solutions, in comparison with nonaggressive boys, but this problem-solving difference was evident only when the boys' main social goals were taken into account. Thus, children's schemas about social goals and outcome expectations can affect their response decisions in the fifth stage of information processing.

Indirect Effects of Schemas on Social Information Processing

Schemas can also have indirect or mediated effects on information processing through their influence on children's expectations for their own behavior and for other's behavior in specific situations. These indirect effects occur because of the associated affect and arousal when the schemas are activated, and because of the schemas' influence on the style and speed of processing (Lochman & Lenhart, 1995; Lochman et al., in press). In research on socially rejected children, Keane and Parrish (1992) found that knowledge of an antagonist's affect influenced nonrejected children's interpretation of the other person's behavior, but that rejected children did not alter their interpretation based on this information. In a related way, schemas about attributes of self and of others, such as aggressiveness or dominance, can produce expectations about the presence or absence of these attributes as individuals prepare to interact with people in specific situations. Lochman and Dodge (1998) assessed aggressive and non-aggressive boys' expectations for their interpersonal behavior before a 4-minute competitive discussion, as well as their perceptions immediately after the interaction. Lochman and Dodge (1998) found that aggressive boys' perceptions of their own aggressive behavior, after live dyadic interactions, were primarily affected by their prior expectations, whereas nonaggressive boys relied more on their actual behavior during the interactions to form their perceptions. These results indicate that the schemas of aggressive boys about their aggressive behavior are strong and compelling, leading the aggressive boys to display cognitive rigidity between their expectations and perceptions. The aggressive boys' perceptions of their behavior, driven by their schemas, were relatively impermeable to actual behavior and were instead heavily governed by the boys' preconceptions. Thus, aggressive children in general, like socially rejected children, are more inflexible at the interpretation phase and may not take relevant new information into account (Lochman & Lenhart, 1995).

Schemas are complex blends of cognition and associated emotion, and as schemas are activated during interactions, they can contribute to the intense levels of affect and arousal that a person can experience in response to a provocative event. Thus, although provocative events produce some emotional and physiological arousal in most children, the intense reactive anger and rage of some individuals can be due to the activation of schemas about the general hostility of others, as well as schemas about the role of others in initiating unjust and unfair conflicts. Emotions have been hypothesized to be the glue between attributions and behavior (Weiner & Graham, 1999) and the adaptational systems that motivate individuals to solve their perceived problems (Smith & Lazarus, 1990). For example, when a child attributes blame for a conflict to another person, the child experiences anger, but when the child has perceived self-responsibility for the problem, the child experiences guilt (Weiner & Graham, 1999). These attribution–emotion linkages can then produce quite different decisions about behavioral responses (e.g., aggression vs. apology, help seeking, nonconfrontation, or compromise). Schemas about accountability and responsibility, with their implications for who receives blame or credit for events, are closely linked to the experience of anger. Accountability appraisals generate "hot" emotional reactions when a provocative person is perceived to act intentionally, unjustly, and in a controllable manner (Smith & Lazarus, 1990). The arousal and emotional reactions in early stages of interactions then serve to flood the information-processing system (Lochman, 1984) and to maintain the hostile attributions and aggressive response style over time during an interaction. Craven (1996) has found that in a laboratory setting, increases in heart rate following a provocation are correlated with increases in hostile attributional biases. This makes it more difficult for the aggressive individual to avoid escalating cycles of aggression and violence. Aggressive children and adolescents are further hampered by schemas and appraisal styles that make them relatively unaware of emotional states associated with vulnerability (e.g., fear, sadness), leading them to overlabel their arousal during frustration or conflict as anger (Lochman & Dodge, 1994).

Aggressive children have an impulsive cognitive style, leading them to spend less time carefully evaluating perceptions and response decisions during interpersonal events. Instead, they rely on reflexive and automatic information processing (Lochman et al., 1981). Schemas can influence aggressive children's overreliance on automatic processing in several ways. Aggressive children can form a belief that it is important to respond quickly to provocative events, rather than carefully evaluate their potential solutions to problems. This belief can form because of the real dangers these children have previously faced within their neighborhood or family setting. However, when the belief is strong, compelling, and impermeable, the children may not easily recognize that contextual differences make the belief less necessary in certain situations (e.g., when at school or with less threatening peers). In addition, because of the internal arousal and emotion activated by schemas about provocation or threat, aggressive children tend to use rapid, automatic processing. Aggressive children's social problem-solving style has been found to become less competent when they are using automatic processing rather than deliberate processing (Lochman, Lampron, & Rabiner, 1989; Rabiner, Lenhart, & Lochman, 1990). When using automatic processing, aggressive boys generate more action-oriented solutions, more help-seeking solutions, and fewer verbal assertion solutions. Therefore, children's schemas can have indirect effects on their appraisals of self and others and on their problem solving by eliciting excessive automatic processing and short-circuiting the children's more competent deliberate processing.

ANGER COPING: A COGNITIVE-BEHAVIORAL INTERVENTION FOR AGGRESSIVE CHILDREN

Based on this social-cognitive model of the cognitive and emotional distortions and deficiencies that aggressive children display, the Anger Coping Program was developed and refined to address core difficulties with emotional and cognitive self-regulation, including anger management, physiological and emotional awareness, perspective training and attribution retraining, and social problem solving. Following the initial development and evaluation of the Anger Control Program (Lochman et al., 1981), the Anger Coping Program described in this book was developed on the basis of further research on these social-cognitive processes. The Anger Coping Program, created for use in school and clinic settings (Lochman et al., 1987; Lochman, FitzGerald, & Whidby, 2000), uses an intervention model that is closely linked to the social-cognitive developmental model that accounts, in part, for the initiation and maintenance of aggressive behavior. In subsequent chapters, we describe practical implementation issues involved in the use of this program in school settings.

CHAPTER 3

♦♦♦

Getting Started with the Anger Coping Program: The Collaborative Roles of Group Leaders and Teachers in Selection and Treatment

♦

James ripped a poster off the wall on the way down to the group room, then Terry tripped Michael so that he cut his lip on a table. While the co-leader took a bleeding and crying Michael to the nurse, James and Anthony got into a shoving match over some smuggled candy and James ripped Anthony's shirt. The group hadn't even started the session yet.

Too frequently, hard-working group leaders are so understandably concerned about what is or is not happening in the group room that matters of generalization become a "hope for the best" affair. Moving children with aggressive externalizing behavior problems out of their respective classrooms and down the hall to the group room, then getting them settled, attentive, and participating, and finally moving them back to the classroom, without a major catastrophe, is a success in itself. Additional concerns associated with training for generalization often become lost.

Yet what is the purpose of all that effort if not to have a positive effect on behavior out of the group room? A young fourth-grade student in a group run by one of the authors once remarked, "I wish this was my classroom, because I do good in here and don't get in no trouble." That child was expressing a training need: "Help me to transfer my functional behaviors in this therapy room to the more critically relevant setting of my classroom." As everyone knows, children are referred to school psychologists and guidance counselors because of their behavior in settings *other than* the group room.

Unquestionably, obtaining insight and skills in the therapy setting is a critical first step, but only a first step. For direct intervention to be useful to the child, a bridge to the problematic setting must be constructed. It is the quality of the collaboration between the group leaders and the classroom teacher that will define the quality of that bridge. Both of these professionals have a critical role to play in the implementation of a meaningful intervention, and neither can ignore or undervalue the contribution of the other. It is for that reason we dedicate this chapter to a discussion of the interdependent roles of group leaders and teachers in the development and implementation of an anger control counseling group.

QUALIFICATIONS AND QUALITIES OF GROUP LEADERS

The program we will discuss was designed as a school-based intervention for use by a trained co-leader team consisting optimally of a counselor and a school psychologist. The involvement of a community mental health professional as a co-leader is also appropriate (Lochman & Wells, 1996). Although busy schedules and tight resources may demand that only a single group leader manage the intervention, a co-leader situation is most advantageous for the following reasons:

1. Two adults in the group room provide a greater sense of personal security for the children and may reduce any anxiety they have concerning their own safety and well-being. It is not unusual for the children to initially "test" the group environment to determine whether it is one that will be characterized by control or lack of control. The visible presence of two adults can help to reduce or alleviate some of these concerns.
2. Co-leaders can divide the group leaders' chores, with one addressing the training and the other concentrating on behavior

management concerns. This issue is discussed in a later section.

3. The addition of a second adult allows the leaders to plan and execute behavioral modeling of the activities or skills for the children to observe. The Anger Coping Program is a skills-based intervention and, as such, draws procedures from effective teaching as well as from counseling. Skills are generally trained using what might be termed a "discuss, observe, rehearse, apply" model, thus allowing the group members to watch the leaders role play the designated skill is a critical feature.

4. The co-leaders can debrief one another following each session to gain additional insight into the progress and direction of the group. Using immediate postsession time to share observations, make training adjustments, and plan strategies is very important to the potential effectiveness of the intervention.

It is highly desirable for at least one of the co-leaders to have had previous supervised experience with school-based therapy/counseling groups. Disruptive, noncompliant, and highly externalizing young children are not the population with whom to begin learning group counseling techniques without supervision! Although a good anger control intervention is comparatively structured and clear with regard to session-to-session activities, there is little substitute for the skills and confidence gained through previous experience in managing a counseling group.

Because the most effective anger control programs are based on a cognitive-behavioral framework that draws heavily on a social-cognitive model of anger arousal (see Lochman & Wells, 1996), it is essential that the group leaders have a strong working foundation in the theoretical underpinnings of the program prior to implementation. In general, the graduate training of school psychologists and guidance counselors is excellent preparation for the group leader's role. Indeed, their individual disciplines and expertise combine well in addressing both selection assessment concerns and the group counseling aspect. However, not all preparation programs place emphasis on working with aggressive children. In lieu of specific graduate course work in cognitive-behavioral theory and intervention techniques, an intense study of the first two chapters of this book, along with selections from "Recommended Further Reading" (found at the end of this book), is highly recommended. Requesting that the local university provide a continuing education opportunity in work with angry, aggressive children can also be very beneficial.

Broadly defined, the primary responsibilities of the group leader in an anger control counseling group are the following:

1. Initiate, design, and cooperate with the classroom teacher, parents, and relevant others in the process of screening and selection of group members.
2. Establish a collaborative relationship with the classroom teacher, and assist that individual in learning and enacting the necessary responsibilities for classroom support of the intervention.
3. Collaborate with the classroom teacher on the determination of behavioral goals for the group members.
4. Obtain informed parental consent; determine and implement the appropriate level of parental involvement in the intervention.
5. Inform and involve the administrator in understanding and enacting his or her role in the intervention.
6. Develop a behavioral management plan for the group setting, including procedures for moving the students in and out of the classroom.
7. Secure the appropriate physical setting and necessary supplies for implementing the program.
8. Conduct the intervention training in accordance with the prescribed procedures.
9. Design and implement appropriate progress monitoring and outcome efficacy assessments.
10. Arrange and conduct booster sessions with the group members following the completion of the intervention.

Let us address the first three critical elements in the group leader's responsibility, as they effectively set the stage for the rest and involve the classroom teacher to a significant extent. The teacher has three important responsibilities in an anger control intervention: (1) participating in screening and selection, (2) collaborating on treatment generalization in the classroom, and (3) evaluating classroom behavioral goal attainment efforts. In this chapter, we examine how the group leader and teacher work together in each of those areas.

SCREENING AND SELECTION OF STUDENTS

Some years ago, a school psychologist was settling his anger control group in for their first meeting, when one of the children asked how it came to be that he was selected for this group. Before the group leader could answer, another boy piped up, "He just asked the teacher who the baddest kids was, and here we are!" That answer, although reduced to its most oversimplified and colloquial elements, was not far off the mark. However, not every aggressive child needs anger control group skills training, and for some it may even be contraindicated. Although the kids may see it as simply identifying the "baddest" pupils, the real process is considerably more complex.

The participation of the teacher in the identification and treatment of students in the anger control group is fundamental to any hope for successful outcomes. Identifying the students who are most likely to benefit from a small-group skills training is the first phase of what will be a collaborative effort between the teacher and the group leaders over the course of many weeks to come. The school psychologist or counselor who perceives that a direct intervention group may be the treatment of choice for some problematic students needs to begin the process in a systematic and thoughtful fashion. The teacher may be ready to merely point out "the baddest kids" and leave the rest to the group leaders, but his or her role goes much beyond that.

An effective anger control program is designed to provide angry, aggressive children with important anger management and problem-solving skills and to prevent progressively more serious conduct problems in later years. Consequently, finding and selecting the children most likely to benefit is paramount. The goal of an effective identification process is the early and reliable identification of children most at risk of later serious antisocial behaviors (Charlebois, LeBlanc, Gagnon, & Larivee, 1994). The term *reliable* is key here. The limits on the time and resources of school personnel make it essential that the process identify children who are at "true risk" rather than those with adequate skills and other protective factors who are merely going through a difficult, time-limited period (known as "false positives").

In addition, the screening and identification process itself must be time- and cost-effective. Procedures that place excessive demands on human hours and school budgets stand little chance of being absorbed into the regular fabric of the education program. Although providing each child at the grade level with a complete psychological evaluation would likely yield adequate data for reliable selection, few if any school psychologists have time for such an assessment. Some manner of middle ground between that option and simply having the teacher rattle off the names of the most problematic children should be adopted. Because of his or her expertise in assessment, the school psychologist should be consulted at each step of this screening process, even if he or she is not a part of the treatment team.

The use of *multiple gating procedures* for the identification of children at high risk for later conduct problems has been advanced by a number of authors (e.g., Loeber & Dishion, 1983; Loeber, Dishion, & Patterson, 1984). These methods use relatively inexpensive ratings as a first "gate" and more sophisticated identification procedures for later gates (Charlebois et al., 1994). This "ever-narrowing gate" process is an effort to both identify those children at true risk and reduce the number of those who may be false positives. A number of models have been examined, including those that utilize teacher-driven ratings (e.g., Sinclair, Del'Homme, & Gonzalez, 1993; Walker et al., 1988), peer and teacher ratings (e.g., Roff, 1986), and parent and teacher ratings (e.g., Whebby et al., 1993). Jones, Sheridan, and Binns (1993) used deficits in early social skills as identifying variables for high-risk children.

A large body of research suggests that economic disadvantage, inadequate parental discipline practices, and early oppositional behavior are among the major risk factors related to later conduct disorders (see Kazdin, 1987a, 1995, for reviews). Specific research on the Anger Coping Program indicates that children with the highest initial level of disruptive-aggressive off-task classroom behavior and with the poorest problem-solving skills have been shown to make the strongest gains (Lochman, Lampron, Burch, & Curry, 1985). An effective multiple gating process must acknowledge these risk factors and marker behaviors and attempt to target the children at highest risk. The multiple gate screening and selection process described here makes significant use of both teachers and parents' observations and ratings of behavior.

Gate 1: Lowest Socioeconomic Group

Because of the strong relationship between low socioeconomic status and a host of later risks (e.g., Attar, Guerra, & Tolan, 1994; Yung & Hammond, 1998), economically disadvantaged districts, or school attendance areas within larger districts with the higher proportions of economically disadvantaged families, should be targeted as the first gate. This is not to say that comparatively well-off school districts do not have children at risk for aggressive behavior; clearly, they do. However, poverty has the capacity to potentiate other risk factors to such a great extent that its role in the selection process cannot be ignored. If there is no clear variation in the socioeconomic status of the student body, then the process should proceed to Gate 2.

Gate 2: Teacher Nominations

At the identified grade level, teacher nominations of pupils who show at least three of the following should be solicited: (1) marked difficulties with interpersonal problem solving and anger management (including interpersonally aggressive and nonaggressive responses), (2) oppositional and disruptive responses to teacher directives, (3) rejection from the more adaptive peer culture, and (4) academic failure or underachievement. A sample Teacher Nomination form is shown in Appendix A.

Our experience has been that some teachers are afraid that nominating a child for consideration will "label" him or her unfairly. Group leaders should provide assurance that the teacher is only suggesting names of students who will go on to be carefully screened later. There is no danger that a child will receive services based only on the ratings at this second gate. To that end, teachers should be advised to err on the side of possible overidentification at this stage. There are a number of other factors to be considered in the nominations:

1. Children whose aggression provides them with high peer status and who do not express any motivation to change should be left out of the nomination process. Often these children are seen as the school bullies, and they may use their aggressive behavior proactively to intimidate, harass, and physically as-

sault other students. These children are a significant source of concern, and their needs—along with those of their victims—should also be addressed by school personnel. Helpful work by Batsche (1998) and Olweus (1993) may provide guidance for such intervention efforts.

2. Avoid inclusion of children who are substantially different from the proposed pool of nominees. For instance, children who are in the same classroom grade but 2 or more years older, as a result of multiple retentions or for other reasons, may be inappropriate because of differing developmental issues. Similarly, aggressive children who are typically withdrawn or who have very fragile self-concepts may be inappropriate for this intervention, as their impulses may become excessively aroused during the role-playing activities (Lochman et al., 1987).

3. Aggressive children who are currently being served in special education programs for those with emotional disabilities should be included if their co-occurring disorders do not (a) provide excessively high stimulation for possible verbal or physical abuse from more aggressive peers or (b) offer the potential for extraordinary behavior management concerns for the group leader.

4. Because of the need to understand the social-cognitive processes involved in the training, pupils in the anger control program should be functioning at, at least, a low average intellectual level.

Gate 3: Teacher Screening Scale

Following informed parental consent, the group leaders should meet with the teacher and assist in the completion of the Teacher Screening Scale (adapted from Dodge & Coie, 1987) for all of the children nominated in Gate 2. This scale is shown in Appendix B. (Parental consent at this step is necessary and proper because a subset of individuals, rather than the entire class, is being assessed.) This scale was selected because of its promising support in research trials and its simplicity and ease of use for larger-scale screenings. However, professionals who trust and have experience with other similar scales should feel free to substitute them. The goal of this stage of the selection process is to establish a hierarchy of need and risk among those children first identified by the teacher.

The Teacher Screening Scale has demonstrated modest promise in the ability to discriminate reactive and proactive aggression patterns. Note that the first three items (single asterisks) are representative of reactive aggression, and the final three items (double asterisks) show proactive patterns. Although the data indicate that teachers typically view aggressive behavior patterns in children as unidimensional (Dodge & Coie, 1987), the two-factor nature of this instrument can prove useful in those cases in which the teacher reports strong ratings in one direction or the other. For example, if a child scores very high on items 10, 11, and 12 and very low on items 1, 2, and 3, the treatment team may want to further assess whether the child would be better suited in a bullying intervention rather than an anger control program. Caution is advised against overinterpretation of the Teacher Screening Scale, however. The lack of adequate research support in an applied setting argues for a very conservative approach. Look for broad, sweeping differences in scores rather than minor variations. The school psychologist's expertise in psychometrics will be most valuable in this analysis.

Comparison of the global ratings on this instrument will give the group leaders and teacher a working hierarchy of children considered in need of anger and aggression management training. Revisiting the initial Gate 2 nomination list with the new data may allow them to move selected children from anger control group consideration to less invasive classroom-level interventions.

Gate 4: Broadband Assessment

The teacher and the parents of each identified child should be asked to complete a broadband behavior checklist. Well-standardized instruments such as the Child Behavior Checklist (CBCL; Achenbach, 1991), the Behavior Assessment System for Children (BASC; Reynolds & Kamphaus, 1992), or other related multidimensional parent/teacher rating instruments should be utilized. The use of multidimensional instrumentation allows for examination of possible co-occurring symptoms, which may lead to additional recommendations for treatment. For instance, the high occurrence of aggression and oppositional behavior among children diagnosed with attention-deficit/hyperactivity disorder (Barkley, 1998) demands that the possibility for the presence of this disability be considered. In this instance, the use of a broadband instrument at this juncture allows the treatment team to look for significant elevations on hyperactivity and attention deficit indices. In addition, studies with children who have conduct problems have reported rates of comorbidity with internalizing difficulties as high as 52% (McConaughy & Skiba, 1993). These findings indicate the necessity to examine the protocols carefully for the existence of all co-occurring problems that may require additional intervention.

Parents should subsequently be contacted and interviewed in order to clarify their responses and gather specific behavioral information. This is an opportune time to begin to understand the strengths and willingness of the parents to participate in the intervention (see section on parent participation in Chapter 4). At this gate, the treatment team is most interested in whether the child is displaying behaviors at home similar to those seen in the school. Issues of setting demand (i.e., differing demands and behavioral expectations between home and school settings) should be taken into account. For instance, it is common for parents who place few compliance demands on their children to be unaware of the noncompliant or oppositional behavior seen at school.

Those children observed by parents and teachers to have significant externalizing behavior problems in both the home and school environments should be identified and considered the first priority for intervention. Children who have been reliably identified as problematic in the school setting but not in the home setting should be included in the second tier of candidates.

Preintervention Individual Assessment

Once the pool of pupils has been identified through the multiple gating process, the treatment team needs to further evaluate their individual characteristics. How much does anger play a part in these pupils' difficulties? What are their current problem-solving competencies? What is the function of their aggressive behavior? For instance, children with highly affective reactive aggression will have intervention needs that are, in many ways, distinct from those of children with lower-affect, proactive aggression levels (Dodge & Coie, 1987). In addition, children with primarily proactive aggression patterns and adequate peer social acceptance tend to view their behavior as less problematic than their more reactive peers and, consequently, may be less motivated to participate in treatment (Lochman, White, & Wayland, 1991). This individual assessment will allow the group leaders to (1) better understand the functional antecedent and consequent events associated with the problematic behavior, (2) individualize the intervention emphases to meet the particular needs of the group, and (3) select out those pupils for whom the intervention may be contraindicated because of their characteristic anger or aggression.

The choice of the assessment instrument or procedure will naturally be guided by the nature of the assessment question. Although an exhaustive description of individual assessment procedures and instruments is beyond the scope of this chapter, a number of excellent resources are available. Lochman, White, and Wayland (1991) have provided a comprehensive discussion of assessment options for use with aggressive children. These authors suggest procedures and instruments for the evaluation of social problem-solving strategies, peer group status, familial/parental functioning, cognitive/academic deficits, and self-concept. Furlong and Smith (1994) review an extensive selection of psychometric measures intended to assess anger, aggression, and/or hostility in children and youth. McMahon and colleagues (McMahon & Estes, 1997; McMahon & Wells, 1998) provide a model of assessment that stresses not only the assessment of the child's behavior per se, but the behavior in interactional contexts of school and home environments. In addition, three scales for the measurement of anger—the Children's Anger Response Checklist (Feindler, Adler, Brooks, & Bhumitra, 1993), the Anger Response Inventory for Children (Tangney, Wagner, Hansbarger, & Gramzow, 1991), and the Children's Inventory of Anger (Nelson & Finch, 2000)—provide useful assessments of anger-related problems and affect.

Pretreatment Authentic Data

In addition to these psychometric data, group leaders at this time should also obtain "authentic" or school record data on the selected group members. These data may include (1) accumulated discipline reports, such as office referrals, detentions, and suspensions, (2) tardy or absentee reports, (3) academically related data, such as homework return rate or other teacher-suggested measures of adaptive classroom skills resulting in a permanent product. This information will serve the dual purpose of helping the group leaders to better understand the actual problems the children are having in school and providing a comparison baseline for posttreatment evaluation. Having a useful, data-based estimate of the relative effectiveness of the intervention is essential to good counseling practice. The preintervention data, psychometric and authentic, can contribute to that assessment effort. (See Chapter 10 for additional discussion on assessing progress.)

Once the group members have been identified, it is now time to assist the teacher to further understand and refine his or her collaborative role in the intervention.

TEACHERS AS TREATMENT COLLABORATORS IN THE CLASSROOM

From a group leader's perspective, the anger control program brings together both *direct* and *indirect* intervention—the group leader working directly with the children in the treatment room and indirectly through the teacher in the classroom. For this combined approach to result in positive outcomes for the children, the group leader and the teacher must have a strong, professional working relationship.

When school psychologists and other supportive services personnel engage in direct intervention efforts, it is not unusual for the child's classroom teacher to be relegated exclusively to the role of clock-watcher, who says to the child once a week: "Time to go to group." Not that this function is unimportant, but it hardly stretches the potential of the classroom teacher to participate in the change process. One of the principal factors that make school-based therapy so viable in comparison with clinic-based therapy is its location in the authentic setting (Coie, Underwood, & Lochman, 1991; Tharinger & Stafford, 1996).

Along with the obvious benefit of ease of access to the population of concern, the potential for generalization offered by conducting treatment in the school is considerable. School is where the children interact with one another and is a major arena for interpersonal aggression. Having ready access to the problematic individuals while they are within the problematic setting provides significant opportunities for creative, collaborative, and potentially generalizable treatment programs.

To upgrade the classroom teacher from "time keeper" to true collaborator, the group leader must take into consideration two pertinent issues: (1) the skill and the willingness of the teacher to become involved in classroom-level interventions and (2) the actual time the teacher has available to participate, given the myriad other responsibilities.

Experience has shown that most teachers are willing—sometimes eager—to assist in the treatment of children in their classrooms. However, it is a rare teacher who will spontaneously *volunteer* to work with a group leader unless the two have collaborated similarly in the past. Typically, the group leader—school psychologist or counselor—must initiate the collaboration.

The literature on school-based consultation is rich with discussions and recommendations for consultants attempting to establish effective working relationships with teachers (see, for example, Brown, Pryzwansky, & Schulte, 1995; Conoley & Conoley, 1992; Marks, 1995). Some related points are addressed here.

Promoting an Egalitarian Relationship

Like a consultation between teachers and supportive services staff members for purely academic problems, the cooperation between teacher and group leader is a collaboration of two professionals, each with his or her own area of expertise. If the group leader attempts to enter this collaboration with the implied message, "I'm here to rescue you from these difficult children," a potentially ruinous hierarchy, consisting of the "Expert Therapist" and the "Inadequate Teacher" may evolve. The capacity for this hierarchy to become firmly entrenched, particularly with new or less-skilled teachers, is significant. When a group leader enters a classroom and hears the teacher say, "Well, guess what *your* kid(s) did today?" then the time has come to reexamine the collaboration.

The group leader needs the teacher as an equal working partner in order to achieve success in the intervention. Communicating respect for the expertise that teachers bring to the collaboration is a critical feature leading to that desired partnership. Among other important skills, the classroom teacher has (1) a knowledge of the course and the nature of the curriculum, (2) instructional abilities, (3) classroom discipline strategies, (4) an understanding of the interpersonal dynamics in the classroom, and (5) a knowledge of his or her own skill and willingness to participate in the intervention. Also important, the teacher has regular access to the child and influence over the child's behavior. The capacity of the classroom teacher to be an effective agent of change should not be underestimated.

Emphasizing Voluntary, Time-Limited Cooperation

Assure teachers that their cooperation is voluntary and that the classroom aspect will be limited to that allowed by their available time and energy. If at all possible, avoid any implication that a "greater authority" (e.g., the principal or a powerful parent) is encouraging or requiring the intervention. This sets up the teacher's role in the intervention as another "duty" that is being observed from above, and few teachers believe they have extra time for more duties. In similar fashion, a group anger management program should not brought to the teacher disguised as some manner of benevolent gift that the teacher has no choice but to accept (e.g., "I'm the school psychologist and I'm here to do you a *really big favor*").

Instead, the most effective collaborations arise logically and systematically out of the authentic situation. Because direct intervention is more "invasive" than indirect—in that the children must be *extracted* from the classroom environment for the treatment—it should be among the last interventions attempted. A pryamidal structure of intervention with a schoolwide discipline plan at the base, working upward toward direct intervention near the top, exemplifies this principle (see Figure 3.1). Has the teacher exhausted all the classroom-level interventions? Should this intervention be directed instead at enhancing teacher skills in an area such as classroom discipline or conflict resolution?

The amount of time the teacher must devote to his or her part of the intervention is a major variable in acceptability (Conoley & Conoley, 1992; Elliott, Witt, Galvin, & Peterson, 1984). Group leaders who themselves have never had responsibility for the day-to-day education of an entire classroom of elementary children may have difficulty understanding a teacher's hesitancy to surrender even small

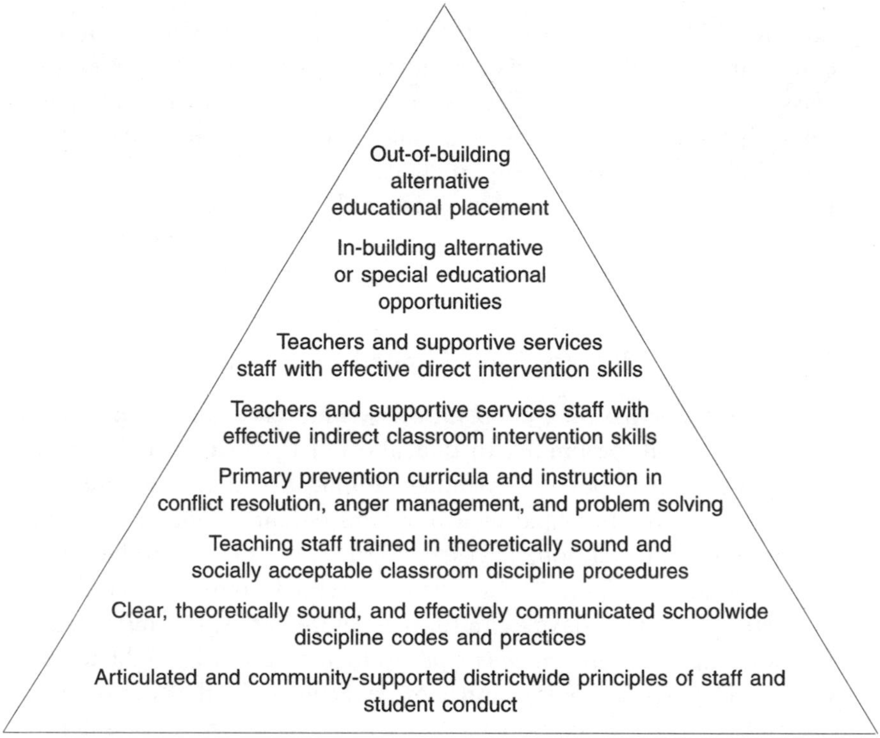

FIGURE 3.1. Pyramid of intervention for angry, aggressive students, with location of anger control program.

amounts of time. While working as a school psychologist, one of us (Larson) was approached by a teacher, who requested that he administer an intelligence and an achievement test to all 32 of her second-grade pupils. Because it was September, she reasoned that the data would be a helpful guide in her instruction as the year progressed. This well-meaning teacher was ignorant of the other demands on the psychologist's time and may not have understood either his initial look of horror or his attempts to gently suggest an alternative strategy.

In similar fashion, nonteaching support personnel must respect classroom teachers' ownership of their available time. An honest estimate, based on experience if possible, should be provided so that teachers can realistically assess their availability to participate. For example, the group leader might say the following:

"In my experience, teachers have found that an extra 10 minutes per day is the average time they have devoted to the Anger Coping Program responsibilities, with perhaps a little more on our meeting day."

Or:

"Well, this is my first group, so I am unsure about what your time commitment might be. Can we see how the first week goes and make any adjustments we feel necessary at our next meeting?"

It is also important to be open to teachers' conclusions about what they can or cannot do. When teachers say, "I'll do *this*, but I don't think I have time to do *that*," they almost always mean it. Trying to persuade a reluctant teacher to agree to additional intervention time creates a genuine danger that he or she may say yes to an unrealistic commitment. Such a collaboration, in which one partner believes that he or she is working too hard, is not a healthy situation for either party.

The Teacher as an Agent for Generalization

Treatment is not only about change, it is about generalization of that change. It is one thing to demonstrate anger management skills in the group room, but it is quite another to do so in the authentic environment of the classroom. Most experienced group leaders working with children who show angry, aggressive externalizing behavior problems in the school setting have anecdotes about failure to transfer or generalize what was supposedly learned in the therapy room. The experience of a group leader believing a student client may now have finally acquired alternative-to-aggression skills, only to find that student fighting before the morning is out, is not an unusual one. Working hard in the treatment room but leaving generalization to chance often yields predictable results:

GROUP LEADER: He teased you and you hit him?
STUDENT: Yeah.

GROUP LEADER: But didn't we just work on that in the group?

STUDENT: Yeah.

GROUP LEADER: And what is the thing to do?

STUDENT: Just walk away or use my self-talk to calm down.

GROUP LEADER: Why didn't you do either of those?

STUDENT: I don't know.

A useful example with which readers may identify is a student learning to drive an automobile. The simulators in the driver's education classes provide an opportunity to enact many of the behaviors necessary for the required skills in the safety of the classroom. It is, however, unimaginable that students would subsequently be handed the car keys without additional effort aimed at getting them to generalize those skills to a "real" situation. "Learner vehicles" with dual breaking systems and giant, cone-lined driving courses are all a part of that generalization effort.

Elliott and Gresham (1991) discussed three classes of generalization: setting generalization, behavior generalization, and time generalization. Setting generalization refers to the child's ability to exhibit a behavior out of the setting in which it was originally trained. For example, if a child has been taught to use self-instruction to control angry outbursts in the training group and then subsequently uses this skill in the classroom, setting generalization has occurred. If a child has learned a problem-solving procedure in the therapy situation and later utilizes that procedure to nonaggressively resolve a problem on the playground, then setting generalization has occurred.

Behavior generalization refers to behavior changes that are related to, but are not the focus of, direct training. For example, a child who was trained to replace aggression with verbal assertion in peer interaction is observed to have also begun to use negotiation strategies. Related behaviors in response to the same problem situation are grouped together under the rubric *functional response class*. Students referred for intervention because of aggressive behavior may have numerous verbally and physically aggressive responses available to them. For instance, a student accused of misbehavior by the teacher might throw a book, knock over a desk, swear at, threaten, or even assault the teacher, particularly if any or all of these responses have led to a positive outcome in the past. All of these behaviors belong to a functional response class. One of the goals of direct intervention, therefore, is to establish and expand the more adaptive functional response class.

Finally, time generalization refers to the ability of the child to maintain the intervention behaviors after the training is discontinued. Behaviors will be maintained to the extent that they continue to be functional and reinforced. Changes that occur during treatment stand a greater likelihood of maintaining or generalizing over time if the reinforcements remain the same (Kazdin, 1982; Martens & Meller, 1990). This finding argues for the use of naturally occurring reinforcers such teacher and peer approval or positive regard ultimately used to replace any more artificial procedures.

There is, however, absolutely no research suggesting, or reason to believe, that skills trained in the group room will transfer or generalize usefully anywhere else—whether to the classroom, the playground, or the neighborhood—without specific generalization guidelines built into the fabric of the intervention. Pupil insight and skill mastery within the setting of the group room are critical prerequisites, but they are only prerequisites. The most important objective—indeed, the raison d'être of the entire effort—is to facilitate the adaptive transfer of the desired skill to the authentic environments of school and home. The mechanism for this to happen cannot be conceived as an afterthought or an add-on; it must be integrated into the structure of the intervention at the onset. Too much is at stake in the lives of these children to rely on the "train and hope" model.

Lochman and Wells (1996) pointed out that children who have a history of noxious behavior in the classroom setting create an expectation on the part of the teacher that the behavior will continue. This creates a self-perpetuating mechanism in which the teacher assumes that a particular child is responsible for any disruptive behavior and may automatically blame the child even in questionable circumstances. The unfairly blamed child then responds in anger and quickly transforms him- or herself from "victim" to "perpetrator," reinforcing the teacher's belief. This insight makes it absolutely essential that the teacher become an active, full partner in the intervention process.

Ensuring that teachers have a sense of ownership in the effort at the outset by involving them systematically in the selection process is the first important step. The next step is to educate them regarding their specific roles. For teachers to take on these roles as true collaborators, it is necessary for them to know on what they are collaborating. Although this seems obvious, it is frequently the case that psychologists and counselors do not share the specifics of the treatment with classroom teachers. It may well be that some supportive service people prefer to mention a certain "mystique" about what happens in the treatment room, or, more likely, it may be that they have never perceived the need to be more forthcoming with teachers. The group leader and the classroom teacher, as a collaborative team, need each other to be as informed as possible about what is happening in the other's environment. Role plays and behavioral rehearsals in the treatment room that are directly related to actual classroom dynamics are more useful to the child than those that are unrelated. Similarly, in the classroom the teacher is more able to accurately observe and reinforce a newly acquired treatment behavior if the teacher knows what to look for and expect.

For teachers of pupils in the anger control program to facilitate this generalization in the authentic environment, it is critical to provide them with an adequate understanding of the goals, objectives, and procedures of the intervention. The following serves as a useful procedure for group leaders in accomplishing this task:

1. Find 30 minutes to 1 hour in the week before the sessions begin when you can gather together all of the teachers in the building who will have students in the Anger Coping Program group. A group meeting is preferable because teachers can share concerns with one another, and it saves time.

2. Provide the teachers with a handout that summarizes the objectives of each session and offers suggestions for facilitating generalization in the classroom (see Appendix C for an example). If the *Anger Coping Video* (Larson, Lochman, & McBride, 1996) is available, it can provide a helpful visual aid for selected sessions.

3. Proceed through the sessions in order, discussing the objectives and soliciting ideas for mutual assistance—for example, "How can we best help one another so that the intervention is most effective? How might this skill be transferred to the classroom setting?"

4. Solicit input from the teachers regarding treatment group

behavior management strategies with the children identified for the intervention. Their knowledge of the children can prove valuable and allow initial meetings to progress more efficiently. For example, knowing ahead of time that Manuel is instantly angered by Jason's chronic teasing about his father, or that Derrick responds very well to adult praise, can be of genuine assistance.

5. Make arrangements to meet with each teacher individually prior to the start of the first group meeting to gather behavioral data for the goal-setting activity.

Now that the teachers have a knowledge of the goals and structure of the treatment and have shared their concerns and ideas, their ability to function collaboratively with the group leader is increased. Our experience is that some teachers will welcome the new challenge and others will be less enthusiastic. Group leaders must always remember that the children were referred initially because their teacher viewed them as problematic, and the children remaining as candidates once the selection process is complete are the *most* problematic. It does not take much imagination to understand why a teacher, besieged with the needs of a classroom full of other children, cannot match the group leaders' enthusiasm in addressing the needs of the most disruptive. As the process moves to the goal-setting interview, patience, support, and understanding will help carry the day.

GOAL ATTAINMENT EVALUATION UTILIZING THE GOAL SHEET PROCEDURE

A central feature of an effective anger control intervention involves the development by the individual group members of classroom behavioral goals. In the program manual contained in Chapter 7, the entirety of the second session is devoted exclusively to instruction and practice in the development and writing of personal behavioral goals. Each subsequent session opens with an evaluation of how the children are progressing toward these goals. Attained goals are replaced with newer ones.

A goal is defined for the group members as meeting the following two criteria:

1. Something you want and are willing to work for.
2. Something that is real and possible for you.

The training involves helping the group members devise classroom goals that address behaviors that are currently problematic but within their ability to alter in a positive direction. Overbroad, ill-defined goals such as, "I will not get into any trouble" are rejected in favor of more specific, behaviorally defined goals such as, "I will remember to ask permission to get out of my desk during seat work time." The goals are written on individual Goal Sheets and delivered to the classroom teacher at the conclusion of each group session.

The group members' goals are the major training link to generalizing behaviors to the authentic setting. The question of whether a group member has or has not attained his or her goal is the sole domain of the classroom teacher who signs the Goal Sheet (Appendix D) at the conclusion of each school day. This makes it essential that each goal, as derived and defined by the child, is clearly expressed and pertinent to teacher concerns. A goal devised by a child that the teacher sees as meaningless or too easy among the child's larger constellation of problematic behaviors will work against both generalization and teacher cooperation. For instance, a child may express a goal of "no fighting in the classroom for at least 4 out of 5 days," only to have the teacher confirm later that historically the child's problem has been at recess and never in the classroom.

The Teacher Interview

To help ensure that the children will be using the Goal Sheet procedure to address classroom behaviors that their teachers agree are problematic, a pregroup conference between group leaders and the classroom teachers is essential. This conference should occur once the final roster of group members has been solidified and before the first meeting. The role of the Goal Sheet in the anger control intervention should be thoroughly explained to the teachers.

> "If you will recall from our previous discussion of the Anger Coping Program curriculum, the children will be learning how to develop personal behavioral goals at our second meeting. This is a very critical aspect of our effort because it serves as one

of the major bridges between what we are doing in the group room and what you are doing in the classroom. To facilitate the children's goal development, it will be helpful for you to give me some guidance regarding the nature of their problems in your classroom. If I understand your concerns, I can more easily help guide the children toward useful, appropriate goals."

Group leaders are urged to familiarize themselves with techniques of behavioral interviewing (e.g., Busse & Beaver, 2000; Kratochwill & Bergan, 1990) and, if necessary, goal development (e.g., Fuchs, 1995; Meichenbaum & Biemiller, 1998). Teachers of children with externalizing behavior problems often have a difficult time expressing their concerns in terms amenable to intervention. "He never does what he is supposed to do, he's always out of his seat, blows up at everything, and he can't keep his hands to himself" expresses the teacher's frustration adequately but provides only minimal guidance for behavioral goal setting. Once teachers have described the problematic behaviors in their own terms, group leaders should encourage them to focus their concerns in a more behaviorally discrete manner.

GROUP LEADER: It certainly sounds like Michael is quite a handful. I am glad we have decided to work together on his problems. You mentioned that he doesn't comply with your directions, hits other children, aggravates the hamster with his pencil, and pushes and shoves in the recess line. Are those the problems of greatest concern to you?

TEACHER: Yes, along with never finishing his seat work in math.

GROUP LEADER: Okay, considering those problem behaviors, when you say that he "doesn't comply with your directions," what do you mean by that? Can you provide me with a typical behavior?

TEACHER: I guess I mean that he is the slowest one in the class to comply with what I want them to do. I'll say, "Take your social studies book out," and 5 minutes later, Michael is still engaged in whatever we were doing previously.

Group leaders should work through the teachers' concerns in such a manner as to acquire a useful behavioral definition of the problem. For example:

"In unstructured settings such as recess, Michael will strike another child with his fist when upset or frustrated an average of
three times per week."

"Michael will have to be told to keep his hands out of the hamster cage an average of once a day."

"Michael gets out of his seat without permission an average of
four times per hour during seat work periods."

Once these topographical descriptions of the behavior are agreed
upon, the group leader should determine which of the behaviors the
teacher believes to be within the ability of the child to self-monitor
and exert some control. *It is important to note that the behaviors
need not of necessity be aggressive or anger-induced to be appropriate
for the goal-setting activity, particularly at the outset.* Aggressive,
externalizing children often have a host of disruptive, poorly social-
ized behaviors that contribute to their overall problematic adjustment
in school. The goals may address not only aggression toward peers,
but social skills with peers, oppositional and disruptive behavior, and
failure to complete various school tasks (Lochman & Wells, 1996).
The objective of the goal-setting activity—again, particularly in the
beginning of the intervention—is to provide the child with an opportunity to move him- or herself in a positive social direction through
his or her own self-control efforts. Because Michael has been referred
to the anger control group to *learn* anger and aggression management, it makes little sense to expect it from him early on. If, however,
in the initial weeks he succeeds in reducing his out-of-seat behavior
during seat work time, this can be viewed by all parties as a positive
social and academic gain. As the training in the group progresses,
those goals should become more directly associated with anger and
aggression management.

GOAL ATTAINMENT EVALUATION USING
THE MODIFIED GOAL ATTAINMENT
SCALING PROCEDURE

Goal attainment scaling (GAS) as a procedure for monitoring progress in behavioral interventions has been widely used in community
mental health programs for nearly 3 decades. The methodology in-

volves (1) identification of a target behavior, (2) an objective description of the desired outcome of the proposed treatment, and (3) the development of three to five descriptions of the target behavior that approximate the desired outcome (Sladeczek, Elliott, Kratochwill, Robertson-Majaanes, & Callan-Stoiber, 2001). This procedure has applications in the Anger Coping Program with teachers who are motivated to spend a little extra time to provide the data. Appendix E provides a model GAS worksheet that we have found useful. With this procedure, the teacher determines a current level of performance relative to the classroom goal that the child has decided upon, develops a series of approximations, and rates the child daily in his or her efforts toward that goal.

For example, assume that the child's goal is stated as follows: "I will not get out of my seat without permission during seat work time." The rating scale is as follows:

0 = Current level of performance, or what the child typically does during this time; the expected level of performance, perhaps 4 to 5 incidences of out-of-seat behavior; this is placed in the middle of the scale.

To the left of the expected level of performance on the scale:

+1 = Improvement over the expected level of performance, perhaps only 2 to 3 incidences

+2 = Much improvement over the expected level of performance, perhaps 0 to 1 incidence

To the right of the expected level of performance on the scale:

−1 = Poorer than the expected level of performance, perhaps 5 to 7 incidences

−2 = Worst possible outcome, much poorer than the expected level of performance, perhaps more than 7 incidences.

These data may then be quantified and charted by the group leaders over time to provide both a formative and summative progress measure of the effects of the intervention relative to the specified classroom goals. Readers interested in further discussion of goal attainment scaling are referred to Kiresuk, Smith, and Cardillo (1994), and for more general issues in outcome measurement, to Ogles, Lambert, and Masters (1996).

With the group members now identified, the teacher provided in-service in the intervention and enlisted as a collaborator, and the goal-setting activity prepared, the group leaders can begin the final preparations for the start of the intervention.

THE TEACHER AS GROUP CO-LEADER

Implementing the anger control group in a small-population classroom for students with emotional/behavioral disabilities can be an efficient and effective way to address some of the children's behavioral problems. In such a scenario, the classroom teacher is an ideal candidate for the role of co-leader in partnership with an experienced school psychologist or counselor.

One of us (Larson) encountered the opportunity for such an arrangement while working as a school psychologist in a large elementary school. Following a presentation to the general faculty on the roles of the school psychologist, including a brief discussion of implementing anger control training, he was contacted by one of the special education teachers. Her classroom was composed of fourth- and fifth-grade students who had been diagnosed with emotional/behavioral disabilities. It was a resource-type classroom, into which various groupings of students came and went during the day, depending on the instructional settings described in their Individualized Education Plans (IEPs).

The teacher approached the school psychologist with concerns regarding a particular group of fourth-grade children whom she saw for a 2-hour block daily for math and science instruction. She described the children as similarly impulsive, quick to anger, and quick to fight. The teacher was concerned because so much of her time was dedicated to physically restraining students or putting herself between a pair of potential combatants that very little math or science was being taught or learned. These patterns of behavior were also carried over into the general education inclusion classes and onto the playground. She wondered whether she could collaborate on an anger control program with her entire classroom of students.

The school psychologist observed the classroom and reviewed the existing assessment information in the special education folders. Clearly, five of the children were a handful and were everything the teacher described them to be. A sixth boy and a single girl, who completed the classroom population, were much more inhibited and withdrawn than the other five. Parental consent for additional assessments were obtained for the five aggressive children. The teachers of the general education inclusion classroom were asked to complete a broadband classroom rating scale on each child, and parents were asked to complete the home version. The resulting data, although somewhat variable among the children and demonstrating some anticipated differences between settings, was supportive of significant externalizing difficulties in the school setting for each child.

Because the students were in special education, an IEP team had to be convened for each student in order to approve the adjustments in the plan for the Anger Coping Program and to provide an alternative instructional setting for the two children who would not be involved. At those meetings the intervention was explained to the parents, and informed consent was obtained.

The classroom teacher had a solid training foundation in behavior modification techniques, but needed to learn the procedures in the Anger Coping Program before the program could begin. Before the start of the school day, the school psychologist helped the classroom teacher to learn the intervention. It was decided that the school psychologist would take the role of the skills trainer while the teacher would take the role of managing group behavior.

This teacher was a truly outstanding co-leader. Her deep knowledge of the children and the skills she learned and applied as a behavior manager within this setting were a perfect complement to the skills of the school psychologist. Although no "publication-ready" behavioral data were obtained on the effectiveness of this intervention, the teacher was clearly pleased with the effects, and a graphing of discipline reports showed a trend in a positive direction. Anecdotal reports from the general education classroom teachers were also encouraging.

When working with a teacher as a co-leader in "ready-made" groups such as described, group leaders should keep the following in mind:

1. For students who are protected under the Individuals with Disabilities Education Act (IDEA), additional approval procedures are required prior to implementation of any behavioral intervention not already defined in the IEPs. This can be a time-consuming task that the teacher may not have anticipated.

2. Be certain that the teacher has cleared his or her schedule for the period of the intervention and knows that it must be maintained for the duration. As busy as most teachers are, it is enticing for them to occasionally double-schedule the time slot for other obligations, knowing that their co-leader will be with the class. Although this may be the innocent move of an overtaxed educator, it can have a disruptive influence on the group.

3. Help the teacher to avoid problems with his or her dual role as sometimes the students' teacher and sometimes the group co-leader. Being able to "take off the teacher's hat and put on the co-leader's hat," leaving any previous interpersonal classroom problems behind, can sometimes be a challenge.

4. Remember that it is ethically irresponsible to involve a child in an intervention for whom an assessment has not indicated a need. Take care not to allow some students to "sit in" on the group only because they happen to be assigned to a particular classroom at the time scheduled for the anger control program. It may indeed be true for some that "it won't hurt them any," but psychological or counseling services are not delivered under such premises. Alternative programming, consistent with the IEP or other educational plan, should be provided.

5. Our experience is that co-leaders can successfully lead a group of as many as seven children. A single leader is advised to limit the group to four or five children.

CHAPTER 4

◆◆◆

Expanding Generalization: Obtaining the Support of Parents, Administrators, and Community Agencies

◆

An effective anger control program is more than just a simple counseling group; it is a broad-based effort to teach the child more adaptive anger and aggression management skills in multiple settings. In the previous chapter, we discussed the critical importance of collaboration with the classroom teacher. We turn now to the subject of parents, school administrators, and others in the larger community who may be selectively brought into the endeavor. As it is with teachers who are collaborating in the intervention, involving other parties as a part of the generalization effort must also be carefully built in at the outset.

WORKING WITH PARENTS

Obtaining Parental Consent

The need to obtain the informed consent of parents or legal guardians prior to delivering direct therapeutic intervention services to children in the school setting is well established within the profession of school psychology (National Association of School Psychologists, 1984). Although school psychologists tend to routinely obtain consent for intervention services, this may not be the practice of other school-based professionals. Because of the comparatively invasive nature of this intervention—assessment and periodic removal from the academic setting over an extended period of weeks—it is our bias that informed consent prior to implementation of the anger control program is essential. Readers are referred to Jacob-Timm and Hartshorne (1998) for a comprehensive discussion of the numerous legal and ethical issues surrounding the subject of informed consent.

Along with reasons associated with ethical and legal mandates, there are additional, more practical considerations for obtaining consent from parents or legal guardians. It is typically the case that the children who have been selected for participation have behavioral difficulties in multiple environments, including the home setting. The process of obtaining informed consent allows the group leaders to further assess and understand how the child's anger and aggression is expressed and managed at home.

Inviting parents or guardians to come into the school to hear an explanation of the program and to provide consent is preferred to mailing or sending a form home with the child. Too frequently, school contacts with parents of disruptive, aggressive children are of a negative nature—for example, a parent is called in by the teacher or principal to account, once again, for his or her child's misbehavior. For that reason, mail from the school may sometimes be intercepted by a child or routinely thrown away unread by a frustrated parent. Moreover, a long, legalistic, information-heavy letter about the intervention may tax the reading skills of some parents, calling into question whether the consent is truly "informed."

Thus, inviting the parent or guardian in for a brief discussion of the intervention can be a welcome break in that pattern. It is very important that the parent or guardian see the anger control program as a positive, proactive feature of the child's total educational experience, rather than a disciplinary, punitive reaction to past misbehavior. Covert or otherwise, the message "We've had it with your kid; we're sending him to the psychologist" should be avoided at all costs. The parents should not come away with the belief that their child is being "sentenced" to a counseling group, but rather that the school is responding to a learning need in much the same way it might for many other skill deficits. Although selection for the group is not necessarily an occasion for celebration, it is an occasion for hope.

A decision must be made as to whether it is most advantageous to hold the parent consent meeting with the group leaders and the classroom teacher all in attendance or with only a single group leader. The former may allow the parent to perceive the intervention as more of a collaborative, schoolwide effort and may encourage his or her participation. Yet for some parents, seated in a room with numerous, often unfamiliar professionals, the experience may be very intimidating and off-putting. On some occasions, the consent meeting may coincide with a regularly scheduled parent–teacher conference. This circumstance may allow for an initial discussion of the intervention with the teacher and the group leader and a subsequent one-on-one continued explanation in the group leader's office.

An informed consent form should include three elements: It should be *knowing, competent,* and *voluntary* (Jacob-Timm & Hartshorne, 1998). *Knowing* consent implies that a parent has a clear understanding of what the group entails for his or her child. What will the child be learning? How and where will this learning take place? Who will be in charge? How much class time will be missed? When will the program be completed? Will an assessment be involved? What will happen if permission is denied?

This communication, like all other communication, both oral and written, must also be in a form understandable to the parent or legal guardian—in lay person's terms and in the parent's dominant language. If no one on the treatment teams is fluent in the parent's language, the services of a trained translator are necessary.

In addition, an informed consent form will provide information about any foreseeable risks associated with the intervention. An effective anger control program does not train a child to engage in any behaviors considered to be dangerous or detrimental to adaptive functioning in either school or home. In our many years with this type of intervention, we have not found any problems of children being singled out or ridiculed for their participation. Careful planning renders the question of lost academic time moot. It is, however, important to address and answer parental concerns regarding any possible "downside."

The issue of confidentiality may also be addressed. In regard to therapeutic counseling of minor children, the laws regarding confidentiality are variable and often unclear from state to state. In regard to whether parents or legal guardians have a "right" to know what

was said within the confines of the counseling group, the conclusions are murky at best. Group leaders will be well served to consult their own state's legal authority. Our experience has been that it is an extremely rare parent who presses this issue. In addition, the nature of the training in a typical anger control program is such that disclosure of private or controversial matters is minimized. It is usually sufficient to assure the parent or legal guardian that he or she will be informed if necessary, in accordance with the state's mandated reporter provisions, and that he or she is always welcome to come in for a conference on the progress of the child in the intervention.

By *competent*, the law means that the individual giving consent is a legal adult who has not been judged incompetent in a legal hearing (Bersoff, 1975). From their experience with special education programming, most school personnel are familiar with the issue of legal authority to provide consent. Group leaders will be well served by adhering to similar guidelines in these instances as well.

Finally, the element *voluntary* means just that: The parents or guardians should not feel coerced in any way to provide their consent for the intervention. The parent's feelings of coercion can be a touchy situation if ignored by the intervention personnel. By bringing the parent or guardian into the school for consent, the school has clearly sent a message: "We've done all this screening and assessment, and we've made up our minds. Now we want you to sign the consent form." Some parents may perceive this as undue pressure by the school. However, if the treatment team has carefully explained why the child was selected and what the intervention entails so that they now meet with a truly "knowing" parent, that pressure is relaxed somewhat. In addition, it is important to assure the parent that nothing dire will happen if he or she refuses consent. The following may be a useful model:

> "It is certainly your right as a concerned parent (guardian) to refuse your consent for this program, and we will honor that right. Please remember, however, that your child was selected for this group because our efforts to help him (her) to this point have not been as successful as we would have liked. Remember also that you can take him (her) out of the group at any time. If you choose not to consent, you can be assured that we will continue working with your child as before in the classroom and

will be open to any additional suggestions you might have. There will absolutely no punitive consequences for your child by your refusal to consent."

A sample consent form is included in Appendix F. This format will work as a mailed consent letter in the event that the parent is unable to come to the school, or, preferably, it can be used as the final signature sheet following an in-person explanation. Schools should modify this sample to meet their own local needs.

Involving Parents in the Intervention

School personnel are often inclined to point their fingers at parents when it comes to attributing causes for the disruptive, aggressive behavior of their young pupils. Given what is known about the possible roles of families in the development of aggression (e.g., the coercive family process work of Patterson and colleagues noted in Chapter 1), that attribution can be substantially accurate in many cases. As noted previously with regard to teachers, parents, too, can hold self-maintaining beliefs with regard to the aggressive behavior of their children, expecting it and even reinforcing it (Lochman & Wells, 1996; Reid & Patterson, 1991).

Consequently, when school psychologists and counselors elect to provide skills training to children, the question arises: How can we provide one set of skills in school, only to have the children go home to learn the polar opposite set of skills? If the parents continue to use aggressive disciplinary procedures, model aggression in their interactions, fail to monitor aggression in sibling problem solving, and do not discourage violent television or video games, isn't the school swimming against an irresistible current?

The positive side to the answer is that if such parents can be persuaded to participate fully in a well-designed, carefully structured parent management training (PMT) program, good things can happen. Patterson (1974, 1982) has demonstrated that training parents to more effectively obtain child compliance, to monitor the child's behavior in and out of school, and to recognize, reinforce, and model prosocial behavior can produce reductions in aggressive behavior. Kazdin and Weisz (1998), in their review of the literature involving aggressive children, concluded that parent management training had significant potential as an intervention, noting that "PMT is one of the best-researched therapy techniques for the treatment of oppositional and aggressive youth" (p. 26).

Yet working with parents of high-risk children in a structured intervention program is not a frequently observed feature of most school offerings (Miller, 1994). Numerous factors mitigate against its ease of incorporation into service delivery options, including work hour restrictions or building availability in the evening, perceived lack of expertise among staff, or funding constraints. In addition, parents who are struggling with the many elements that have been found to characterized the coercive parenting family, such as poverty, drug and alcohol abuse, divorce, and criminality (Reid & Patterson, 1991) also struggle with the organizational and motivational processes needed for active engagement in training. Even with expensive incentives such as monetary stipends, child care, transportation, snacks or even dinner, attendance rates of less than 50% are typical (Lochman & Wells, 1996; Prinz & Miller, 1994).

In spite of the logistical, motivational, and budgetary obstructions, the potential benefits of parent training are too promising to simply write off as unfeasible. Practitioners who are able to acquire the financial and other resources necessary to construct and implement a parent training program are encouraged to go forward. Collaboration with a community agency that may already have a funding or logistical structure in place is an option to be considered.

Miller (1994), in her review of family-based interventions for angry, aggressive children, identified six critical parental competencies for training:

1. Tracking, labeling, and pinpointing. Parents should be taught to more effectively monitor their children's behavior, to avoid global descriptions of the behavior ("He never does what I ask him to do") and to monitor antecedent and consequent events around misbehavior.
2. Emphasis on positive child behavior. Parents should be taught to recognize and attend to prosocial behavior in their children with appropriate social reinforcers.
3. Giving appropriate compliance commands. The importance of clear, unambiguous communication from the parent to the child should be emphasized and the necessary skills trained.

4. Nonphysical discipline. Parents should be introduced to and trained in a variety of discipline procedures, such as time-out, response cost, and ignoring.
5. Effective communication. Learning how to listen actively, empathize, resolve conflicts, and cope with personal feelings of anger or depression cued by child misbehavior should be trained.
6. Troubleshooting and generalization. Parents should be taught how to apply skills across different settings and to increase collaborative efforts with the school.

Numerous existing programs from which to select or adapt are available (e.g., Barkley, 1997; Forehand & McMahon, 1981). Lochman and Wells (1996) discussed the implementation of a parent training component with the Coping Power Program in Durham, North Carolina. This intervention consisted of 18 sessions with the parents of children who were receiving treatment in an expanded version of the Anger Coping Program. The parent program, adapted from existing social learning theory models, included the training of skills in helping parents identify target behaviors for their children, rewarding appropriate behavior, establishing developmentally appropriate expectations, applying effective consequences, managing behavior outside the home, and establishing effective communication structures.

Webster-Stratton and her colleagues (Webster-Stratton, 1989a, 1989b, 1992; Webster-Stratton, Kolpacoff, & Hollinsworth, 1988) have developed a videotape program for use with parents of children with conduct problems, entitled *The Parents and Children Series: A Comprehensive Course Divided into Four Programs* (Webster-Stratton, 1989a). The program is based on a cognitive social learning model (Webster-Stratton et al., 1988) and trains parents in a wide range of parenting skill areas, including play behaviors, use of praise, limit setting, and alternative discipline techniques. The procedure makes primary use of prerecorded vignettes that stimulate group discussion among parents. Generalization for parents is approached through the use of "homework" handouts concerning a number of topics (e.g., monitoring commands, establishing household rules) and behavioral assignments, all contained in a parent workbook. Selected subsets of this program, such as the limit setting and alternative discipline procedures, may be particularly worthwhile.

The Office of School Psychological Services in the Milwaukee (Wisconsin) Public Schools authorized the creation of a parent training program for use in the school setting entitled *Parent to Parent: A Video-Augmented Training Program for the Prevention of Aggressive Behavior in Young Children* (Larson & McBride, 1993). Drawing from the work of Patterson and colleagues (Patterson, 1982; Patterson et al., 1975) the program is designed to train parents to monitor their children's behavior, to recognize and reinforce prosocial behavior, to use self-instruction to guide their own parenting efforts, and to model and teach problem solving.

For practitioners who decide to include a formal parent management training component, the following caveats from our experiences may prove helpful:

1. Plan well ahead of time, as there will be a budgetary impact. Know the budget cycle of the school board, and time your request accordingly. Seek outside funding from grant sources such as those that may be found at state or federal school safety programs or other funding pools for high-risk students. Remember that these children are at risk for myriad problems—academic failure, special education placement, substance abuse, delinquency—so there are numerous opportunities for grants under prevention initiatives. For assistance with these grants, contact the state public education consultant for school psychology or school guidance counseling. Money may also be available locally through police department community outreach funds, private foundations, or local civic organizations.

2. It is often helpful to hold the meeting(s) in a central location in the community, rather than in the school building. Many parents of children with disruptive behavior problems have developed a hostile bias against or fear of school-related meetings of almost any sort. Moving the parent training off school grounds will tend to decrease those concerns somewhat and may have a positive effect on attendance. In addition, such a move may save some of the costs associated with security, custodial services, and utilities that come with opening a school building in the evening. Church meeting halls, community centers, and other facilities available to nonprofit organizations work very well and are often available free of charge or at a very reasonable cost. Public transportation routes, particularly in urban areas, must be considered in planning the location.

3. Meet with the parents personally to explain the reasons for the group; do not count on a phone call, mailed letter, or a note sent home with the child. The "personal touch" puts a human face on the entire effort and sends the message that this is not just another school event to be avoided. Call and remind the parents on the day of the first meeting, and help them deal with any impediments to attending, if necessary.

4. Have sufficient resources to cover transportation, child care, snacks, and a stipend. The parents should suffer no out-of-pocket expenses. The stipend should be over and above the expenses for transportation and child care. It should be provided in an envelope at the conclusion of each session, in cash if possible, to cover "miscellaneous expenses" incurred by the parent in coming to the group. The authors have found $10 per session to be adequate. School boards may balk at this budget item, but our experience with grocery vouchers, school bookstore vouchers, and not stipend at all, has demonstrated the power of simple cash to keep parents—especially those of limited financial resources—returning for additional sessions.

5. Under no circumstances should school personnel conduct a parent training group on a "volunteer" basis, that is, not as official employees of the school board. Whether or not the group leader is being paid for the off-hours parent training, there should be direct, written, informed administrative approval. Continued liability coverage by the school board for a possible malpractice lawsuit must be ensured when any school personnel are working in nonschool settings during off-hours with occasionally troubled adult clients. Personal coverage by the practitioner's own carrier is also recommended.

Clearly, not everyone who is able to implement an anger control intervention in the school will also be able to implement such parent training programs as have been described. However, it is certainly not a foregone conclusion that limited parent involvement will translate into poor outcomes for the children. Indeed, most of the positive program effects discussed in a review of the anger management research were obtained without a significant parent training component (see Feindler & Scalley, 1999; Lochman & Wells, 1996).

At a minimal level, parent involvement can be secured during the assessment and consent processes. Beyond that, an effective anger control program should have a continuing parent communication procedure. The Anger Coping Program described in Chapter 7 utilizes three parent letters that are sent at prescribed intervals during the program to reach this goal (see Appendices I and J). These letters inform the parents about what their children are learning in the group, make suggestions as to how they can reinforce what their children are learning, and offer a tear-off portion for feedback to the treatment team. The letters are not intended as a substitute intervention vehicle to alter parents' behavior in a manner similar to parent management training. In fact, it is likely that they have little or no effect on parent behavior beyond providing simple information and inviting input. They are, however, a positive communication from the school regarding the efforts of the child, and the value of such communication should not be underestimated. In addition, the letters function as a record of efforts to involve parents in the treatment of the child, a record that may be important should a referral for special education be made in the future.

Although the daily interactions in the home environments of many chronically aggressive children may continue to play a negative role in their behavior, it is nevertheless important for school personnel to distinguish between an *attribution* for the development and maintenance of aggressive behavior and an *excuse* for not doing something about it. Simply because the parents have been unable or unwilling to make substantive changes in their child-rearing practices, school personnel should not assume permission to throw up their hands in surrender. Children can and must learn to discriminate their behavior according to particular environments, to recognize and enact socially adaptive behavior in multiple settings: "What behavioral choices are in my best interest at home? At the playground? In church? At the mall? On the street? At school?" Clearly, they differ.

Among the major responsibilities of educators is to help children make the important adaptation to the school environment, regardless of what they may be learning elsewhere. Although aggressive posturing and behavior *may be* adaptive in some settings, it is generally maladaptive in the school setting, and children must learn socially adaptive replacement behaviors if they are to find success. Parental support and involvement are important and very helpful in this process, but their absence does not condemn the intervention effort to failure by any means.

THE ROLE OF ADMINISTRATORS

As discussed earlier, an effective anger control program is not reduced to an isolated hour in the child's week, but permeates throughout the system of his or her educational experience. What is happening outside the group room is every bit as critical as what is happening inside. Consequently, all the critical subsystems within the school that interact with the child should be involved at some level, including administrative discipline.

Referring students to the administrator for incidences of aggressive behavior has been shown to be one of the most frequently selected interventions in the school setting (Larson, 1993). The fact that being sent to be scolded or otherwise disciplined by the principal is still as employed as frequently as it is can be considered a testament to how far some schools have yet to go in understanding chronic childhood anger and aggression. The principal has limited choices: talking with the child about the behavior, holding the child out of class for a while, calling the parents in or suspending the child to home, or, in numerous states, applying some form of corporal punishment. None of these interventions has been demonstrated to have a lasting effect on chronically aggressive behavior. Indeed, in comparing states that do and do not allow it, the use of corporal punishment has been shown to be positively related to higher rates of student interpersonal aggression (Hyman et al., 1997).

In many cases, it is the very children already identified for the anger control group that the principal sees day in and day out for one form of misbehavior or another, making it likely that this administrator will have a serious interest in the intervention effort. Consequently, it is advantageous for the treatment team to open the lines of communication with the administrator early in the process. An informational meeting, in which the names of the pupils who will be in the group is shared and a brief explanation of the nature of the training is given, is important. Principals are often justifiably concerned about parents, so the process of securing parental consent and any plans for parent training should also be shared.

Principals, like teachers and other lay personnel, may misunderstand and misjudge the relative efficiency and effectiveness of anger and aggression management training. Knowing that a child is receiving "extra services" but still having behavior problems can possibly cause the principal to become even more frustrated with the child. Group leaders may have to remind the administrator that the program is a long-term effort and that change will come slowly and in small, rather than grandly observable, ways. An adjusted plan for administrative discipline of the children in the group—particularly with principals prone to the use of suspension—should be worked out. For example:

1. Explain the "Hassle Log" (see Appendix H) procedure and provide the principal with a small stack of these forms. This may prove very useful to both parties should a discipline situation arise.
2. Encourage the principal to reference the anger control training and to use a problem-solving strategy during any conference with the child in regard to his or her behavior.
3. When the principal has some disciplinary latitude with regard to a particular offense, ask that he or she refrain from administering out-of-school suspension so that the child will be available for group.

In addition:

4. Urge the principal to "catch 'em being good" at frequent intervals. Remarks such as "I hear you are doing well on your goals" or "You must be proud of the positive changes you are making" may not only reinforce the child but also begin to change what may have become a soured relationship between the two.
5. Invite the principal to sit in on one of the groups. It is respectful of the group members' privacy to ask their permission first, however.
6. Finally, keep in regular contact with the principal, sharing the children's progress and keeping their positive efforts and accomplishments on the principal's "front burner."

THE ROLE OF THE COMMUNITY

As has been emphasized, the Anger Coping Program addresses the needs of the child as a member of the school, family, and community systems by bringing members of those system into the intervention effort. To this point, discussion has centered on the roles of the teachers, parents, and administrators. Let us turn now to that of the community outside the school. As a preface to this discussion, it is important for group leaders to be aware of potential confidentiality issues when communicating with nonschool or nonfamily members about the treatment of minor children (see Jacob-Timm & Hartshorne, 1998, for a discussion). When in doubt, it is always prudent to secure from the parent or legal guardian written permission for release of information to outside agencies, particularly if it involves the release of specific assessment or behavioral data. Most school districts have such release forms available. In addition, it is respectful of the privacy of the children to involve them in any decision to communicate about their treatment to nonschool or nonfamily personnel.

One of the first considerations in attempting to involve the community is an assessment of what it may have to offer. Admittedly, when working with younger elementary school children, the impact that community agencies such as the police and juvenile courts may have is often minimized. Yet even with students as young as 9 or 10 years of age, the possibility that they may have ongoing police or court involvement should not be ignored. If the school has a police liaison officer who has had contact with any of the group members, he or she can be a useful addition to the generalization effort. It thus becomes important to provide a brief in-service training session or explanation to the officer ahead of time and offer suggestions as to how he or she might assist by referencing the anger control skills during any interactions with the group members.

For a child who is on juvenile court probation, a letter or phone call informing the probation officer of the child's involvement in the anger control program at school will most often be well received. The officer may want to meet with the group leader to discuss the training, though given their often overwhelmingly large caseloads, this would be unusual. It is our experience that probation officers are grateful for anything the school may be doing to facilitate improved problem solving among children in their caseloads.

In addition, many communities sponsor after-school programs and activities that can serve as rich environments for practicing and reinforcing the skills learned in the anger control group. With written parental consent (and permission from the child), the group leaders may wish to inform the activity supervisors of the student's participation in the group and make simple, easily performed suggestions for the after-school supervisors. These may take the form of (1) recognizing and reinforcing prosocial, cooperative behavior, (2) encouraging the use of problem-solving strategies, and (3) recognizing and reinforcing anger management efforts.

When a group member is receiving concurrent psychological treatment through a private clinic, on either a family or individual basis, communication with the professional treating the child is warranted. Following both parties' receipt of an informed, written release of information from the parent, it is often useful to exchange information regarding general treatment methodologies (e.g., cognitive-behavioral, client-centered, family systems, etc.), treatment goals, and current progress. The group leaders may find themselves able to function as generalization aides for work that may be happening in out-of-school therapy, just as the therapist may similarly assist the in-school effort. Once again, it is respectful of the privacy of group members to seek their permission before communicating with outside professionals.

Now that the groundwork for the involvement of teachers, parents, and other individuals has been laid, we turn to final preparations for the initial group meeting.

CHAPTER 5

◆◆◆

Preparing for the First Meeting: Procedures to Implement and Pitfalls to Avoid

◆

In this chapter we discuss some of the "nuts and bolts" issues involved in making the group function as smoothly as possible. The insights and suggestions in this chapter are drawn not only from our own many experiences conducting the Anger Coping Program and related interventions, but also from those of the numerous interns whom we have supervised and from practitioner feedback at advanced training sessions. Clearly, there are many "wheels" that have already been invented by many people, and it is our hope to spare the reader the task of having to invent them all over again.

THE GROUP ROOM

To say that available space to run counseling groups in school buildings is a prized commodity may be an understatement. Those who have been asked to conduct psychological or counseling services in converted storage closets, book rooms, stage areas, and old basement staff lounges ("What's that smell?") know of what we speak. It often seems that supportive service personnel are at the bottom of the room and space allocation hierarchy in the school building. Even when a decent office exists, the act of trying to stuff a group of children into a space best fitted for individual services invites the kind of trouble so frequently associated with overcrowding—further intensified because of the presenting concerns of externalizing behavior problems. All the desire and know-how needed to conduct therapy groups is useless if there is no place to implement them.

Ideally, the group area should be large enough for four to seven children to be seated, with abundant space between them to discourage physical contact. In addition, the space should provide enough "moving around" area to conduct activities and role plays. School personnel without their own large office space may have to become creative. The following locales have been utilized by previous anger control groups and are noted here as suggestions:

- A classroom emptied for a weekly library, art, or physical education period
- The gym or a multipurpose room, with the use of portable dividers in a corner area
- The stage area
- The cafeteria
- The conference room
- The nurse's office

A good group room setup is thoughtfully designed in much the same way that a good classroom is arranged. The goals in both cases are to control the antecedent conditions that may encourage discipline problems and provide those conditions that encourage self-control and participation. Group leaders are urged to approach this ecological aspect seriously and systematically, as it can either pay off or punish in the end. They should carefully examine the available space with an eye toward creating a counseling environment best suited for the encouragement of self-control.

To the extent possible, the room should be a very low stimulus environment. This may mean placing distracting toys, games, and other items out of sight during the period the group is in session. Drapes or blinds should be drawn to reduce focus on what is happening outside. Portable room dividers can serve a very useful purpose toward these ends, providing both a space delimitation and a shield for potentially distracting stimuli. Ambient noise is more difficult to control in a school building, but avoiding meeting times that overlap with recess and other times when there is noise caused by student movement can help somewhat. One intern, conducting her second group in a noisy part of a building, played classical music at low volume. She reported that the effect on the children was uncertain, but that the effect on her was positive and significant.

Experience has shown that the most advantageous seating arrangement has the chairs placed in a semicircle, with one leader at the opening of the circle and the other seated midway between the group members. Once again, ample space between the chairs is important to discourage the impulse for even playful physical contact. Taped lines on the floor for the chair spacing can be useful and can give the group members a sense of each having his or her own area.

Some groups have been successfully positioned around a large table, but such an arrangement has distinct drawbacks. Tables in therapy situations have traditionally been seen as offering a "psychological protection" for the client that is absent when the chair is in the open. (Note that the TV talk show host sits behind a desk while his or her guests do not.) Whether or not this notion has merit, the table does offer abundant unmonitored space beneath for kicking and other mischief. In addition, table surfaces can too easily turn into head rests, game boards, or drums, creating another distraction for everyone. Group leaders who find themselves forced to use a table will have to provide the children with additional structure and training to help them avoid the attendant problems.

BEHAVIORAL MANAGEMENT STRATEGIES

Group counseling with highly externalizing children provides an opportunity for them to learn how to function adaptively in a controlled, safe, rule-governed environment. They have been assessed and found to have behavior repertoires that are incompatible with many of the stimulus demands of the classroom. The group environment creates a mini-world, with stimulus demands that are designed to be more easily learned and assimilated. Along with the anger management and problem-solving skills that are a part of the training, the child in the anger control group also learns how to modify and adapt his or her behavior to meet the demands of the setting. In doing so, the child gains experience and practice in the controlled setting that can be used in efforts at generalization to the classroom setting. For this to happen, a systematic program of external consequences and self-management strategies must be designed by the group leaders.

The key phrase is "simple but effective." Complex, elegantly conceived behavioral plans may look good on paper, but they often wither under the reality of fast-paced group interactions and competing stimuli for the group leader's attention. Skill training is difficult enough without the additional stress of trying to remember and implement an overcomplicated management strategy that may be more intrusive than effective. Our experience has been that groups work most effectively when the management strategy stays in the background, operating beneath the skills training and not competing with it for the group members' attention. When everything grinds to a halt so that the group leader can engage in a dispute with a child about whether points (or stickers or candy) were or were not earned, then the management strategy has intruded too far into the training.

In the Anger Coping Program, a simple operant reinforcement strategy and a response cost strategy work in tandem. Simply stated, the group members are reinforced for targeted behaviors to be increased and experience negative consequences for targeted behaviors to be decreased. These targeted behaviors are kept few in number and make intuitive sense in the framework of a smoothly running group.

Recall that *positive reinforcement* is the presentation of a consequence immediately following a behavior that increases the likelihood of that behavior being repeated (Kazdin, 2001). If the consequence has no effect on the preceding behavior, it is not a reinforcer. For example, a child may be presented with a sticker following a desirable behavior, but if the probability of that behavior's being repeated does not increase, then the sticker is not a reinforcer. Similarly, a child may be presented with a smile or a "high five" following a desirable behavior, and if the probability of the behavior increases, then the consequence (smile, high five) is a reinforcer. It is not unusual to hear inexperienced therapists complain that a child "is not responding to the positive reinforcement." That complaint is a contradiction in terms: If it is positive reinforcement, *by definition* it must have an effect on the behavior. The therapist most likely has not identified a true positive reinforcer

POINTS AND STRIKES

Points

In the Anger Coping Program, we have found that desirable behavior is best encouraged and strengthened through the use of a point-based token system. A token system uses tokens or "points" that serve as conditioned reinforcers exchangeable for more tangible backup reinforcers (Miltenberger, 1997). The basic components of a token system include identifying the following:

1. The tokens that will be used as conditioned reinforcers
2. The desirable target behavior that the group leaders want to strengthen
3. The backup reinforcers or tangibles that will be exchanged for the tokens
4. A reinforcement schedule for delivery of the tokens

Simply acknowledging and recording points in a designated spiral notebook as they are earned is the least obtrusive manner to award the tokens (e.g., "I like the way you helped Raymond solve that problem, Hector. That's a point"). Group leaders can pair verbal praise with a nonverbal signal, such as a touch of the leader's nose, and eventually fade the verbal praise to the extent desired. Approaches that are more complex—and thus somewhat more open to problems—include using manipulatives such as poker chips or play money as tokens. Our experience with manipulative tokens is that they often give rise to intrusive counting and comparing among the group members. On the other hand, many veteran therapists have skillfully used manipulative tokens effectively in other contexts and can easily adapt the procedure to the Anger Coping Program.

Regardless of the procedure, leaders should maintain a visible running total on a poster board or other medium. The group members will always be interested in how many points they have earned. It is recommended that leaders not waste valuable group time entering these figures but instead do it themselves ahead of time. (However, one of our interns had the children enter their own totals weekly onto a computer spreadsheet program with reported success.)

A final caveat: As with any behavioral intervention, if the procedure works, use it; if it doesn't, change it. Don't adhere doggedly to an ineffective behavior management approach just because it was the one that seemed appropriate at the beginning. Monitor the effects and make adjustments as necessary.

In the Anger Coping Program, group members typically can earn points for the following:

1. *Smooth transition from class to group room.* This is an oft-overlooked but important element, in that it serves the dual purpose of setting the proper behavioral tone for the initiation of the day's work and prevents difficulties with other school personnel who may be encountered on the journey to the group room. We have found this important enough to encourage leaders to actually practice the transition with the children prior to the first group meeting.

2. *Cooperation and participation in group.* This allows the group leaders to reinforce targeted group behaviors that they wish to increase. Active participation, cooperating with others, ignoring another's misbehavior, and positive leadership can be immediately reinforced. In Session 1, the group members are asked to identify positive behaviors to be encouraged. Providing the opportunity for group members to have a true voice in the establishment of the rules of behavior allows them to assume a level of ownership of group behavioral norms and minimizes future adult–child power struggles (Lochman et al., 2000).

3. *Signed Goal Sheet brought to group.* Group members need to remember to bring the sheets on which they have written their weekly goals (see Session 2), and this is a task that often requires considerable assistance from adults. Providing a point incentive is a part of this effort.

4. *Excused absence points.* We have found that granting 2 or 3 points gratis if a group member is forced to miss a meeting for an excused reason avoids the unhappiness that comes with falling too far behind the others in point totals.

5. *Smooth transition back into the classroom.* This is always appreciated by teachers, and the points are awarded by the group leader as observed following each session. The criteria for earning transition points to and from the classroom should be should be collaboratively devised with the teacher and fully explained to the group members.

The point system serves the dual purpose of reinforcing desirable behavior and providing an opportunity for the group members to learn to manage delayed gratification. We have found that having a time set aside for exchanging points for tangible backup reinforcers approximately every fifth session maximizes the value of the system. Group leaders should acquire an array of tangibles such as pencils, pens, notebooks, and other teacher-approved items for "purchase" at these times. Our experience has been that school personnel are often quite willing to donate these items to the cause; as an alternative, larger department store chains and fast food restaurants rarely need little more than a request on school letterhead to provide free-of-charge items or gift certificates. Group leaders are advised to be certain to obtain school and parental approval for all tangible reinforcers, however. A final "grand prize"—such as a pizza party or popcorn and movie—contingent on the cumulative group total as determined by the leaders, is often very well received and encourages positive peer support for points earned.

An additional note regarding points: Group leaders should be alert to variations in individual behavioral baselines among the children. For example, some children are skilled vocal participants, and if "positive verbal participation" is a criterion for a point, such children are capable of accruing a skewed number of points. Use the point system to help each child grow from his or her current skill level. In other words, avoid overreinforcing those children who already have the requisite skills to earn them while underreinforcing those who have fewer skills. Leaders should keep a flexible "bar" and raise or lower it according to their own clinical judgment to bring the group along with as much parity as possible.

Strikes

Working in tandem with the point system is a response cost procedure (Kazdin, 2001) known in the Anger Coping Program as "strikes." In response cost, the contingent negative behaviors are identified and the individual loses access to a reinforcing condition upon their presentation. Removing access to a favorite toy in response to misbehavior is a common example of response cost. In the Anger Coping Program, the group members are allowed three chances to engage in undesirable behavior at the outset of each meeting (three strikes) before losing the opportunity to stay in the group for the day (the reinforcer). The criteria for losing a strike are decided by the group at the first meeting and are generally some form of a "negative opposite" of the positive points discussed earlier (e.g., disruptive behavior, aggression, teasing, noncompliance, etc.). Once again, it is important to fully engage the group members in the discussion of strikes so that they have the same sense of ownership as they do with the point system.

The group leader is the final and unassailable arbiter of whether a strike is called. Leaders are advised not to engage in a power struggle with a transgressing child. If the child violates the rule, state the violation in a matter-of-fact tone and call the strike. Avoid excessive warnings such as "Jason, I'm telling you for the last time. If you do that again, I will call a strike on you."

Of course, leaders should make an effort to keep their own irritation and anger under control at all times, using the strike as feedback rather than an expression of exasperation. At the outset, in particular, it is important to be consistent, predictable, and clear. Gently but firmly calling strikes as they occur early on in the training can pay dividends later. As noted by Lochman et al. (2000), "This early 'detoxification' of corrective feedback helps defuse aggressive children's tendencies to overpersonalize adult feedback and respond with oppositional or challenging behavior" (pp. 66–67).

The use of manipulatives to keep an accounting of strikes is recommended so that the group member is visually assisted in the effort to monitor his or her own behavior. Group leaders are left to their own creative devices. Previous successful procedures include the following:

1. Place three pencils in a cup in front of each child, pulling one for each strike.
2. Place three playing cards or three strips of tape on the floor in front of each child and remove one for each strike.
3. Write each child's name on a chalkboard, place three checks beside each name, and erase one check for each strike.

If the child has three strikes called, that child should be escorted back to the classroom. Under no circumstances should the child be able to negotiate the option to remain with the group for that day (although it is our experience that most will try). Leaders should always remember that an aversive consequence for one child is a social learning opportunity for the others: They are watching to see what happens. Occasionally, the calling of the third strike will provoke the child to anger or upset. In such a case, if the child needs time to calm down before returning to class, he or she should be escorted to a neutral, nonstimulating third area, such as the administrator's office. Never return an upset, angry child to the classroom.

Group leaders should avoid the inclination to co-mingle the points and strikes by offering a point to those who do not have any strikes called for the entire session. Leaders should provide points for the observed expression of desirable behavior, not just for the absence of undesirable behavior. A child may sit stoically and pout for an entire session, not disrupting, but surely not engaging in desirable behavior worthy of reinforcement.

DIFFICULT CASES

Some children with entrenched oppositional or highly volatile behaviors may struggle with the points and strikes system and provide the leaders with a genuine behavior management challenge. If the leaders find that after two or three sessions, a particular child has been an extraordinary management problem and disruptive to the group process, action must be taken. Ranging from the least to the most intrusive, the following are options to consider:

1. Confer with the child individually to determine whether there are some minor changes that can be made to accommodate him or her. Sometimes ecological issues, such as chair placement, fear of another member, or fear of being called on can stimulate misbehavior. Occasionally, some children are so frightened that they will be called upon to speak that they will misbehave to keep that possibility at bay. Assuring the child that he or she will not be pressured into participation unwillingly can often address this problem. Consider the function of the misbehavior. Is the child trying to avoid or acquire something? Is the child misbehaving so that he or she will be returned to a preferred setting? Is the attention that comes with misbehaving reinforcing to the child?

2. Bring influential others into the problem, such as parents, teachers, an administrator, or another favored adult. Encourage their vocal and enthusiastic support of the child's appropriate behavior in the group setting. Consider a weekly "report card" to a favored adult.

3. Draw up an individual behavioral contract (e.g., Kazdin, 2001) that identifies the specific behaviors to be increased or eliminated and the consequences that will follow. For some children, more

frequent and more powerful reinforcers that go beyond those available to other group members may be necessary. Any concerns by the other group members about perceived unfairness should be addressed in the context of understanding individual differences.

4. Remove the child from the group altogether. Some children are simply not emotionally, developmentally, or behaviorally ready for a highly stimulating, interactive group therapy experience. Indeed, such an experience may be contraindicated, as it may contribute to the child's problem behavior rather than addressing it. Once other efforts have been exhausted, do not hesitate to remove the child and seek an alternative intervention. This course of action, although unfortunate, is certainly much preferred over, as one inexperienced therapist recalled, "hoping each group day that the kid will be absent from school."

USE OF VIDEO

A major portion of the Anger Coping Program is given to addressing deficient problem-solving skills among the group members. This is accomplished by teaching a stepwise model of problem identification, solution generation, and consequence prediction. In the latter sessions, the major vehicle for this learning is the production of videotaped scenarios for which the group members write, rehearse, and tape their own conflict situations for later viewing and analysis. Well before these sessions, it is recommended that the group leaders take time to secure a camera and videocassette recorder/television, as they are often in great demand in some schools. In addition, those who may be unfamiliar with the mechanics of videotape recording are advised to take time to become comfortable with the technology. A headache prevented is one more that does not have be suffered.

To assist in the learning of the concepts in the Anger Coping Program, we have produced a video guide for each session. This video provides training hints for group leaders and in-session models for the children to watch and emulate. Information on how to acquire the video may be obtained by contacting either of us (see addresses at the end of Chapter 8).

The following chapter will acquaint the reader with the outcome research for the Anger Coping Program and for its sister intervention, the Coping Power Program.

CHAPTER 6

◆◆◆

Outcome Research Results for the Anger Coping Program and the Coping Power Program

◆

There have recently been efforts to identify empirically supported treatments and prevention programs for a variety of types of developmental psychopathology, including externalizing conduct problems in children. Kazdin and Weisz (1998) have identified three groups of promising treatments for children with externalizing behavior problems. In addition to parent training (Patterson et al., 1992) and multisystemic therapy (Henggeler, Melton, & Smith, 1992), cognitive problem-solving skills training approaches have been found to produce significant reductions in aggressive and antisocial behavior. As part of a task force on effective psychosocial interventions, Brestan and Eyberg (1998) reviewed the intervention research on children with conduct problems and concluded that the Anger Coping Program was a promising cognitive-behavioral intervention for children with aggressive behavior problems. Similarly, Smith, Larson, DeBaryshe, and Salzman (2000) conducted a meta-analysis of anger management programs for children and youth and concluded that the Anger Coping Program was among the few with both strong design and research support. In this chapter we review the empirical evidence supporting the effectiveness of the Anger Coping Program and describe the Coping Power Program, which is currently being examined in several outcome research studies.

ANGER COPING OUTCOME RESEARCH

Empirical Evidence for the Anger Coping Program

A preliminary uncontrolled study of a school-based Anger Control Program for 12 aggressive children in the second and third grades showed significant posttreatment reductions in teacher-reported aggressive behavior and trends for reductions in teacher checklist ratings of acting-out behavior (Lochman et al., 1981). These improvements in children's aggressive behavior were accompanied by increases in teachers' daily ratings of children's on-task behavior in the classroom. All of the children were African American and lived in single-family homes in a low-income urban neighborhood. The children met with a graduate student therapist twice a week for 12 sessions. These findings spurred a programmatic series of subsequent studies comparing the further-refined Anger Coping Program to alternative interventions and untreated control conditions (Lochman, 1990).

In a subsequent study, 76 aggressive boys from 8 elementary schools were randomly assigned to anger coping (AC), goal setting (GS), Anger Coping plus goal setting (AC + GS), or untreated control (UC) groups (Lochman, Burch, Curry, & Lampron, 1984). The boys were identified as aggressive based on teacher checklist ratings. The boys were in the fourth through the sixth grades, and 53% were African American and 47% were White. They participated in a 12-week Anger Coping group program, based on the earlier Anger Control Program. The boys met in weekly group sessions, lasting 45 to 60 minutes, in their elementary schools. Groups were co-led by university-based project staff (psychologists, social workers, psychology interns) and school counselors based at each school. Goal setting was conceptualized as a minimal treatment condition, and included eight group sessions in which the boys set weekly goals for classroom behaviors and received contingent reinforcements for goal attainment. In comparison with the UC and GS conditions, aggressive boys in the anger coping cells (AC, AC + GS) displayed less parent-reported aggressive behavior, had lower rates in independent observers' time-sampled ratings of the boys' disruptive classroom behavior, and tended to have higher levels of self-esteem at posttreatment. The addition of a goal-setting component, in the AC + GS group, tended to enhance the treatment effects of the program (Lochman et al., 1984), indicating that behavioral goal setting can increase the generalization of cognitive-behavioral intervention effects. Boys in the AC group who had the greatest reductions in parent-rated aggression were those who initially had higher levels of peer rejection, more comorbid internalizing symptoms, and the poorest problem-solving skills (Lochman et al., 1985). The last-mentioned variable was a particularly important predictor of treatment effectiveness, because boys with the poorest social problem-solving skills in the UC condition were likely to have increasingly higher levels of aggressive behavior by the end of the school year.

The effects of the Anger Coping Program have been found to be augmented by the use of an 18-session version of the program, in comparison with the earlier 12-session version (Lochman, 1985). In this quasi-experimental study, 22 teacher-identified aggressive children were included in an 18-session version of the Anger Coping Program (with more emphasis on perspective taking, role playing, and more problem solving about anger-provoking situations) and were compared with the boys who had been in the 12-session program in the Lochman et al. (1984) study. With the longer 18-session program, aggressive boys displayed significantly greater improvement in on-task behavior and greater reduction in passive off-task behavior, illustrating the need for longer intervention periods for children with chronic acting-out behavior problems.

However, in two other studies of the effects of variations in delivery of the Anger Coping Program, the addition of a five-session teacher consultation component (Lochman, Lampron, Gemmer, Harris, & Wycoff, 1989) and a self-instruction training component focusing on academic tasks (Lochman & Curry, 1986) did not enhance intervention effects. Lochman, Lampron, Gemmer, et al. (1989) had randomly assigned 32 children (average age = 11 years) to anger coping, anger coping plus teacher consultation, or to an untreated control condition. Lochman and Curry (1986) assigned 20 teacher-identified aggressive boys (average age = 10 years, 3 months) either to anger coping or to anger coping plus self-instruction training. In both studies, the school-based groups lasted for 18 weekly sessions, and the boys in the anger coping conditions displayed reductions in parent-rated aggression (Lochman & Curry, 1986), reductions in teacher-rated aggression (Lochman, Lampron, Gemmer, et al., 1989), improvements in perceived social competence and in self-esteem (Lochman & Curry, 1986; Lochman, Lampron, Gemmer, et al.,

1989), and reductions in off-task classroom behavior (Lochman & Curry, 1986; Lochman, Lampron, Gemmer, et al., 1989). The Lochman, Lampron, Gemmer, et al. (1989) findings, in comparison with an untreated control condition, replicated the earlier positive effects for the Anger Coping Program evident in the Lochman et al. (1984) study.

In another study of child characteristics that predict intervention outcomes, Lochman, Coie, Underwood, and Terry (1993) found that a social relations program that included anger coping and social skills training components had a significant impact at postintervention and at a 1-year follow-up with aggressive–rejected fourth-grade children, but not with rejected-only children. Relative to control conditions, the intervention outcomes with aggressive–rejected children were reductions in peer-rated and teacher-rated aggressive behavior. This study involved an African American sample from an inner-city area. The result indicated that the intervention was successful because it appeared to influence the mediator variables associated with children's aggressive behavior, but did not influence mediator variables associated with nonaggressive peer rejection.

In addition to the consistent findings from this series of studies indicating that the Anger Coping Program can produce reductions in children's aggression in the home and school settings at the end of intervention, and the Lochman, Coie, et al. (1993) finding that an Anger Coping Program with social skill training components can lead to sustained improvement at a 1-year follow-up, two other studies have examined the follow-up effects of the Anger Coping Program. Lochman and Lampron (1988) conducted a partial follow-up of the Lochman et al. (1984) sample in four of the eight schools. In the follow-up sample, 21 boys had been included in the Anger Coping Program and 10 had been in the untreated control condition. When children's classroom behavior was examined at a 7-month follow-up, the boys in the Anger Coping Program had significantly improved levels of independently observed on-task classroom behavior and significant reductions in passive off-task behavior.

At a 3-year follow-up when the boys were 15 years old on average, those who had received the Anger Coping Program training ($N = 31$) exhibited lower levels of marijuana and drug involvement, lower rates of alcohol use, and had maintained their increases in self-esteem and problem-solving skills (Lochman, 1992), in comparison with those in an untreated control condition (N = 52). Boys who were followed up were highly similar in baseline measures of peer aggression nominations and social status ratings to boys who were not available for follow-up. These results indicate that the Anger Coping Program produced long-term maintenance of social-cognitive gains and important prevention effects on adolescent substance use. Boys in the Anger Coping Program functioning in these domains were within the range of a nonaggressive comparison group (N = 62), indicating the clinical significance of these positive effects. However, boys in the Anger Coping Program did not have significant reductions in delinquent behavior at follow-up, and their reductions in independently observed off-task behavior and parent-rated aggression were maintained only for a subset of boys who had received a brief six-session booster intervention for themselves and their parents in the school year following their initial anger coping group. Thus, across multiple controlled intervention studies, this child-centered cognitive-behavioral intervention reduced children's disruptive behaviors immediately after treatment and provided important preventive effects on adolescent substance use. Booster interventions in subsequent years may lead to less dissipation of treatment effects on children's overtly aggressive-disruptive behavior.

Effects of the Dissemination of the Anger Coping Program

The next stage of intervention research with the Anger Coping Program assesses the program's impact when it is conducted in the field by trained school personnel, rather than by the program developer's trained staff. In this dissemination phase, program developers provide training to school staff and assist with the evaluation, but the program is completely implemented by school staff. As part of a Safe Schools grant, the Wake County (North Carolina) Public School System provided anger coping training to all of the school psychologists and school counselors in the system (Lochman et al., 1998). The training consisted of three full-day workshop training sessions in the spring and summer prior to the implementation of the program, monthly 2-hour large-group consultation sessions during the implementation of the program, and two telephone "hot-line" hours per week during the implementation of the program. The ongoing consultation and hot-line hours were believed to be essential in assisting staff in successfully handling both routine and unexpected problems encountered by school staff during the implementation of the program. Each group was co-led by a school counselor and a school psychologist, and four to six children were typically assigned to each group. Groups began in the fall of the school year and continued through the spring.

Children were identified for inclusion in the Anger Coping Program on the basis of referral from regular education teachers, who selected them based on high rates of physically and verbally aggressive behavior, and of disruptive classroom behavior. Children in self-contained special education classes were not included in the groups, but mainstreamed special education students were eligible. Forty-one anger coping groups were begun at 40 elementary schools, providing service to 200 aggressive children. Pre–post self-report data were obtained from 161 students. Post data were not obtained from students who moved from their schools ($N = 11$) or from students who could not be assessed by the end of the school year ($N = 28$). Because of the limited resources available to pursue nonreturned measures, the rates of completion of pre–post teacher data ($N = 119$) and of parent data ($N = 51$) were lower.

The 161 students with at least partial post data had an average age of 9.8 years, ranging in age from 8 to 12 years. One hundred fifty of these children were male, and 11 were female. Eighty-one were of minority racial status (primarily African American). Forty-six percent of these children received free or reduced-cost lunches, indicating a relatively high rate of low-income children. Forty-one percent were receiving special education services (35 had a learning disability, 7 had a behavioral or emotional handicap, 13 were academically gifted, 11 had other, health-related, problems).

The design of this evaluation consisted of pre–post assessment of children selected for intervention without a control group. However, multiple sources of information about the children's behavior and social competency were obtained to "triangulate" the effects and reduce the likelihood that changes would be simply due to a single-source bias or to artifacts of measuring. A 1-year follow-up of children's academic progress was also performed.

The pre–post analyses indicated that the Anger Coping Program had effects on the relevant mediating variables that should have been affected by the program (Lochman et al., 1998). Children in the anger coping groups displayed significant improvements in their ability to generate competent solutions to social problems, on a measure involving vignettes of hypothetical social problems with peers, teachers, and parents. By postintervention, they evidenced a higher rate of verbal assertion, compromise, and bargaining strategies. They also showed a reduction in their rate of irrelevant problem solutions, indicating that they had improved their cause–effect reasoning in social situations. This reduction in irrelevant problem solutions parallels one of the problem-solving outcomes found in the earlier 3-year follow-up study of anger coping outcomes (Lochman, 1992) and indicates that the problem-solving training in the Anger Coping Program appears to be producing an anticipated effect.

Children in the anger coping groups also showed significant improvements in self-reports and teacher reports of their social competence. Teachers rated the children as being better able to calm down when upset, to recognize their feelings, to handle conflict in more adaptive ways, to cooperate with peers, and to interact in fair ways with peers. The children themselves, on a measure of perceived competence, perceived that they had become more competent in their interactions with peers and more accepted by their peers.

These changes in the children's social competence and social-cognitive skills were accompanied by positive improvements in the children's behavior. Parents reported that the children's externalizing problem behaviors had declined by postintervention, and teachers' ratings indicated that the children's social problems and attention problems had decreased. Teachers reported that 85% of the children displayed at least some reduction in aggressive and disruptive behaviors. Because parents also rated the children as having significant reductions in attention problems, the Anger Coping Program appears to assist children in better focusing their attention in appropriate ways at home and at school. These changes in attentional control may have partially mediated the reductions in externalizing behavior problems, as indicated by the significant correlation between these change scores.

The children's academic achievement was assessed by a state-created achievement measure. The children included in the Anger Coping Program had a 12% improvement at the 1-year follow-up in their rates of grade-level achievement in mathematics and reading, and this improvement was significantly higher than the systemwide improvement rate over the same time period. These children were also found to have a significantly lower rate of increase in school suspensions than was evident for other children their age in this school system. The academic gains at the 1-year follow-up suggest that the children's improved behaviors by the end of the intervention may have contributed to their improved attention and motivation in their class work, which may in turn have led to increased academic achievement. The relative improvement in their school suspension rate suggests that the children's behavioral improvements had generalized over time.

COPING POWER PROGRAM AND OUTCOMES

Coping Power Child and Parent Components

The Coping Power Program (Lochman, in press; Lochman & Wells, 1996) is a lengthier, multicomponent version of the Anger Coping Program designed to enhance outcome effects and to provide for stronger maintenance of gains over time. The Coping Power Program (CPP) has added sessions to the basic Anger Coping Program framework to create a CPP Child Component (for a total of 33 group sessions), addressing additional substantive areas such as emotional awareness, relaxation training, social skills enhancement, positive social and personal goals, and dealing with peer pressure. The Coping Power Child Component program addresses the social-cognitive deficits identified in prior studies. The Coping Power Child Component focuses on (1) establishing group rules and contingent reinforcement, (2) using self-statements, relaxation, and distraction techniques to cope with anger arousal, (3) identifying problems and social perspective taking with pictured and actual social problems situations, (4) generating alternative solutions and considering the consequences of alternative solutions to social problems, (5) viewing modeling videotapes of children becoming aware of physiological arousal when angry, using self-statements ("Stop! Think! What should I do?"), and using the complete set of problem-solving skills with social problems, (6) the children planning and making their own videotape of inhibitory self-statements and social problem solving with problems of their own choice, (7) enhancing social skills, involving methods of entering new peer groups and using positive peer networks (focus on negotiations and cooperation in structured and unstructured interactions with peers), and (8) coping with peer pressure.

Other elements of the CPP Child Component include regular individual sessions, which take place monthly between a child and one of the group leaders and are designed to increase individualized generalization of the program content to the children's actual social situations. The individual sessions are used primarily for monitoring and reinforcing children's attainment of classroom and social behavior goals (e.g., avoiding fights with peers, resisting peer pressure) and for coping with specific attributional biases and social problem-solving deficiencies the children have had in recent social conflicts with peers, teachers, or parents. The individual sessions can also be important in helping to create productive, positive working relationships between each of the children and the group leaders, thus enhancing the positive reinforcement value of the adult group leader. Periodic case-centered consultation is also provided to the teachers of children who are making some progress in group sessions but who are still having recurrent behavior problems at school.

The Coping Power Program also has a CPP Parent Component, which is designed to be integrated with the CPP Child Component and to cover the same 15- to 18-month period of time. The CPP Parent Component consists of 16 parent group sessions. Parents meet in groups of 10 to 12 parents or parent dyads with two co-leaders. Assertive attempts are made to include both mothers and fathers in parent groups. For some sessions, the school counselor can also join the leaders in presenting material relevant to parental involvement in the school.

The content of the CPP Parent Component is derived from social learning theory-based parent training programs developed and evaluated by prominent clinician-researchers in the field of child aggression (Forehand & McMahon, 1981; Patterson et al., 1975). Over the course of the 16 sessions, parents learn skills for (1) identifying prosocial and disruptive behavioral targets in their children, using specific operational terms, (2) rewarding appropriate child behaviors, (3) giving effective instructions and establishing age-appropriate rules and expectations for their children in the home, (4) applying effective consequences to negative child behaviors, (5) managing child behavior outside the home, and (6) establishing ongoing family communication structures in the home (such as weekly family meetings).

In addition to these "standard" parenting skills, parents in this project also learn skills that support the social-cognitive and problem-solving skills that the children learn in the CPP Child Component. These parent skills are introduced at the same time that the respective child skills are introduced, so that parents and children can work together at home on what they are learning. For example, parents learn to set up homework support structures and to reinforce organizational skills around homework completion as children are learning organization skills in the CPP Child Component. Parents also learn techniques for managing sibling conflict in the home as children are addressing peer and sibling conflict resolution skills in the group. Finally, parents learn to apply the problem-solving model to family problem solving so that the problem-solving skills learned by children in the group will be prompted and reinforced within the family context. Some children who have participated in the children's group (i.e., those who were brought with their parents because of a lack of baby-sitting at home) attend the parent group on family problem solving after they have learned the problem-solving model approximately halfway through the children's group. These children and their parents role play the problem-solving skills in parent group, practicing these skills themselves and modeling them for the other parents.

A final section of the CPP Parent Component includes sessions on stress management for parents. Part of the rationale for this is to help parents learn to remain calm and in control during stressful or irritating disciplinary interactions with their children. Parents also receive stipends for their attendance at the parent group meetings. Thus, the CPP Parent Component addresses the mediating factors of parental engagement and children's social-cognitive processes.

Parents are informed of the skills their children are working on in their sessions and are encouraged to facilitate and reinforce the children's use of these new skills. The CPP Parent Component also includes periodic individual contacts with the parents through home visits and telephone calls to promote generalization of the skills learned.

Empirical Evidence for the Coping Power Program

Four grant-funded studies are currently in process to examine the efficacy of the Coping Power Program, and initial analyses have been obtained in two of these studies. In the first of these studies (Lochman, in press; Lochman & Wells, 1999a), 183 boys who had high rates of teacher-rated aggression in fourth or fifth grades were randomly assigned to a school-based Coping Power Child Component, to a combination Coping Power Program including both child and parent components, or to an untreated control condition. Intervention took place over 2 academic years (fourth and fifth grades for some children, fifth and sixth grades for others). Initial outcome analyses indicate that the coping power intervention has had broad effects at postintervention and at a 1-year follow-up on boys' social competence, social information processing, locus of control, temperament, and aggressive behavior, and on parents' parenting practices, anger, and marital relationships. Teachers reported that significant behavioral improvements were evident by midintervention, and parents rated children in the intervention groups, in comparison with children in the control group, as being significantly less aggressive after entering middle school. In analyses of the 1-year follow-up assessment for the first of the two cohorts, most of these effects were maintained. The behavioral gains were maintained most strongly for children who had been in the condition with the combined parent and child components. Most intervention effects, especially in the arena of children's social competence, social information processing, and school behavior were apparent in both intervention cells, indicating the direct influence of the child intervention. However, certain effects, such as parents' sense of efficacy and satisfaction with their parenting, aspects of their marital relationship, and reductions in children's aggressive behavior in the home at follow-up, were evident only in the combined intervention cell, indicating the importance of multicomponent interventions impacting both children's social-cognitive processes and parents' parenting practices. Notably, the highest-risk children displayed a significant reduction in alcohol use at the 1-year follow-up. These results indicate that the CPP intervention had produced substantial change on a range of factors, which would be expected to reduce these boys' future risk for substance abuse, and some of these effects are moderated by the boys' initial risk (or aggression) levels. The results also indicated that parent training can provide significant additive effects to the child intervention in reducing boys' overt externalizing behavior.

The second ongoing study of the Coping Power Program is examining whether the effects of the Coping Power Program, offered as an indicated prevention intervention for targeted high-risk aggressive children, can be enhanced by combining the indicated intervention with an universal prevention intervention randomly offered to half of the fifth-grade teachers and the parents of the students in these classrooms. Indicated preventive interventions are targeted at high-risk individuals, such as aggressive schoolchildren, and universal preventive interventions are provided to all individuals within a certain population, such as all fifth-grade children in a classroom. The universal intervention in this study consists of in-service training for teachers and large-scale parent meetings for all parents of children in universal intervention classrooms. The sample consists of 245 aggressive male and female fourth-grade students who were randomly assigned to one of four conditions: indicated intervention + universal intervention (II + UI), indicated intervention + universal control (II + UC), indicated control + universal intervention (IC + UI), and indicated control + universal control (IC + UC). Intervention began in the fall of the fifth-grade year. Midintervention analyses with the aggressive children indicated that both the universal and indicated interventions produce significant effects on children's social competence and behavior and on parents' positive involvement with their children (Lochman & Wells, 1999b). Initial analyses of postintervention effects, comparing intervention to control conditions, indicate that the combined CPP indicated and universal interventions produce lower rates of substance use, lower teacher-rated aggression, lower expectations of children that aggression will work, higher perceived social and academic competence by children, and lower levels of anger. The CPP indicated intervention by itself produces reduced ratings of parent-rated proactive aggression, lower level of activity by children, better teacher-rated peer acceptance of target children, and increased parental supportiveness. The universal intervention by itself produces lower levels of fearlessness in children and better teacher-rated peer acceptance of target children.

Other ongoing grant-funded studies of the Coping Power Program will determine the effects of a follow-up booster intervention and of teacher consultation and training. A controlled study of the dissemination of the Coping Power Program to a new community is also being conducted.

CONCLUSION

Overall, these results support the efficacy of the Anger Coping Program and of the related Coping Power Program. These programs produce immediate postintervention effects on children's aggressive behavior at home and at school and on their social competence and social-cognitive skills. The programs' effects on social-cognitive processes have been maintained through a 3-year follow-up, and their effects on children's behavioral problems have been maintained through at least 1 year. The Anger Coping and Coping Power Programs have produced significant reductions in children's substance abuse and have notable preventive effects in this area of negative adolescent outcomes. Booster interventions in subsequent years appear to be important in sustaining children's behavioral improvements. This series of outcome studies indicates the value of using these interventions in school-based settings to reduce the conduct problems of preadolescent children.

In addition to the inclusion of booster programs in subsequent years, other possible methods for enhancing the effectiveness of the Anger Coping Program, and of related cognitive-behavioral programs for aggressive children, have been suggested (Lochman et al., 2001). First, group leaders have to be sensitive to negative group processes and to possible iatrogenic (treatment-caused) effects that can occur when group members reinforce each other's deviant beliefs (e.g., Dishion & Andrews, 1995). In regard to selecting group members, we believe that the potential for creating a productive group increases when group members have at least some motivation for working on their anger management difficulties and when the group contains at least some group members who can be solid peer models of how to enact more competent verbal assertion and negotiation strategies. During the course of the intervention, a positive group process can be enhanced by maintaining clear rules and consequences for group behavior, by reinforcing children for positive, prosocial behaviors outside the group, by transferring a child from group to individual intervention when necessary, and by developing positive therapeutic bonds between group leaders and the children.

Second, as noted in Chapter 3, intervention research indicates that cognitive-behavioral interventions with aggressive children produce broader positive effects and better maintenance of behavioral improvements over time if they address both children's social-cognitive processes and parents' parenting practices than do interventions that focus on children or parents alone (e.g., Kazdin, Siegel, & Bass, 1992; Webster-Stratton & Hammond, 1997). Interventions that have both child and parent components can address a wider set of risk and protective factors than interventions with single components (Lochman, 2000a). Preventive interventions for children at high risk for early-starting conduct problems can address the children's school context and academic skills, as well as social competence and parenting skills, across multiple years from elementary school through early high school (Conduct Problems Prevention Research Group, 1992, 1999a, 1999b).

Third, the anger coping intervention should be individualized in several ways (Lochman, 2000b). Even though there is a guiding social-cognitive model indicating the targeted goals for this structured intervention, the intervention should be adapted to address the specific social-cognitive deficits and strengths of the specific aggressive children being helped. As we learn more about meaningful subtypes of aggressive children (e.g., Dodge et al., 1997), we can generate individualized treatment plans that emphasize certain aspects of the Anger Coping Program more than others for particular children. In addition, the Anger Coping Program can be flexibly delivered by adjusting the structured protocol to meet emerging clinical issues. When children begin discussing a current or recently encountered social problem, group leaders can respond by shifting to a problem-solving set, and modeling and reinforcing problem-solving skills directly, rather than rigidly sticking to all of the planned activities for the day. It is critical that group leaders keep the overall objectives of the programs in mind, so that their flexible responses can still have a direct, strategic impact on the targeted social-cognitive difficulties of the children in their groups.

The following chapter presents the Anger Coping Program, with its complete manual for implementation and group leader guidelines.

CHAPTER 7

◆◆◆

The Anger Coping Program Manual

◆

What follows in this chapter is the complete, updated text of the Anger Coping Program, including new individual session-by-session "notes" and helpful hints for the group leaders. This newest iteration of the intervention is closely adapted from earlier manuals found in Lochman et al. (1987) and Lochman, FitzGerald, and Whidby (1999).

The term *session* is used in this manual, but this should not be confused with *meeting*. "Sessions" contain the goals and objectives to be met, but very often multiple "meeting" times are required in order to have the group ready to move on. Group leaders should concentrate on developing skills, without undue concern about the time required, and avoid rushing the curriculum. For instance, scheduling an additional meeting time each week in order to "finish early" is highly discouraged. It is much better to extend the intervention further into the school year, maintaining the support and learning over time. In addition, there is no set number of minutes for a group meeting, but we have found that a minimum of 45 minutes per week is necessary to accomplish a reasonable amount of training, given the time needed for transitions.

As leaders become familiar with the entire manual, it will become clear that flexibility and clinical judgment are important components. Very few "scripts" are presented that detail everything the leader should say or the children should do. Rather, objectives and training guidelines compose the bulk of what follows, and leaders are left to adapt them to the individual training experience. Most of the answers to "What should I do?" or "Did I do this correctly?" can be found within the domains of common sense and clinical experience. Maintaining clear, useful case notes at the conclusion of each meeting and engaging in active co-leader debriefing will be immeasurably helpful.

- ◆ What went well, what did not, and do we know why?
- ◆ What did we learn about the group dynamics and individual members that will assist us next time?
- ◆ Are we following our behavior management program as designed? Does it need to be adjusted?
- ◆ Are we ready to move on to the next session, or is more time needed on the current objectives?

The following manual assumes that the group leaders have read the preceding chapters of this book thoroughly, wherein much information for a successful group experience can be found.

SESSION 1. INTRODUCTION AND GROUP RULES

Group Leaders' Notes

Have the group leaders:

- ◆ Completed all assessments?
- ◆ Secured informed parental consents?
- ◆ Consulted with classroom teacher(s) to establish a collaborative effort?
- ◆ Informed administrator(s) of the purpose and the members of the group?
- ◆ Prepared a behavioral management plan?
- ◆ Discussed and/or rehearsed transition behaviors with group members? (see Appendix G)

During this session, it is important to convey the purpose of the group, set up rules and structure, have the members and leaders become familiar and fairly relaxed with each other, and begin to focus on perceptual and thinking processes. This may be difficult to accomplish in one session. As with all of the following sessions, *it is not necessary that all objectives for a session actually be completed within one session;* instead, an uncompleted objective can be carried over to the following session. Our experience is that such carryover is more often the rule than the exception. Leaders should be more concerned with skill development than with any need to adhere to a lockstep schedule. As in most therapy with children, it is important to make the experience enjoyable. Solid pregroup preparation increases that likelihood, as do plenty of smiles, verbal praises, and (we have found) a candy treat at the conclusion.

Materials

A ball for pass-the-ball

Session Content

Objective 1. Present Group Purpose and Structure

A. Present the group as a way to learn anger control or self-control, or use some other key words or phrase that can be a descriptive slogan of sorts. You may want to discuss how people in general sometimes have problems controlling their anger, or their tempers, moving toward the specific kinds of problems these children have. Encourage group members to volunteer examples of problems with anger control.

B. Issue a statement about the time, frequency, and number of meetings for the group program and give a preview of some of the activities.

C. State the need for group rules and invite the group members to suggest rules they think will be important. Areas to include are confidentiality, physical contact, paying attention and participating, yelling, and so on. It is helpful to write the rules on poster paper or something that can be displayed each session.

D. Discuss the group behavioral contingency system, both for rewards and response costs. Offering the opportunity to earn and lose *points* during the group session, which can later be exchanged for a tangible reward or activity, generally works well (see Chapter 5). Leaders may give some kind of token during group activities for good participation, such as checkers or pick-up sticks, which can be accumulated to earn a point. Similarly, the leaders can call *strikes*, which can also be accumulated to lose a point and may lead to a time-out if necessary. Points can also be accumulated by the group as a whole to earn a group reward, such as special treats or an activity of the members' choosing. Some permanent means of record keeping for points may also be needed.

Objective 2. Get Acquainted

Make sure all group members and leaders know each other by name. If these people are new to each other, a quick means of introduction is to play a pass-the-ball game, with each member holding a ball in turn until that person can name the person to his or her right.

Objective 3. Focus on Individual Perceptual Processes

A. Play the pass-the-ball game with each person having to name something the same (e.g., "We're both boys") and something different (e.g., "He's taller") about the person who threw the ball to him or her. Continue until each member has had a turn.
B. Leaders will have picked out one *DUSO* (American Guidance Service, 2001) or *Second Step* (Committee for Children, 2001)-type stimulus picture, which will be shown to the group but not discussed. Give the instruction that each member is to describe what he or she sees happening in the picture, putting the description on tape. Have the tape recorder in a location away from the group, and give each member a turn. After all have recorded, have the group listen to the tape and then discuss: Did they all see the same things? What was similar and what was different about what they saw? Was there one right way to see the picture?

Alternate procedure. Record the group members' responses to the stimulus picture individually in a meeting prior to the first group session and have the tape ready to play. This is particularly recommended for groups with only one leader.

Provide Positive Feedback and Optional Free Time

Have each group member identify one positive thing about him- or herself and/or one positive thing about another group member. Try to avoid compliments about clothing. Model appropriate compliments as necessary. Following this activity, tally the points earned during the session. Members earning at least 1 point may be given free playtime if the schedule allows. Leaders should use this time to observe for possible conflicts and assist the members in using "problem solving in action." Reinforce prosocial behavior as observed (sharing, resolving conflict appropriately.)

Note. It may be that some or all of the members will get excited or upset during some of the sessions to come. It is very important throughout the rest of the sessions that the leaders take necessary steps to see that the children are returned to the classroom in a "cooled down" state. Free time or low-key structured play can serve this purpose well. The addition of "transition points" added for appropriate classroom return behavior may be useful, and teachers will be grateful.

Leaders: Debrief and Complete Case Notes

◆

SESSION 2. UNDERSTANDING AND WRITING GOALS

Group Leaders' Notes

This session begins a process that continues throughout the Anger Coping Program and that enhances the transfer of the treatment effects into the classroom. Goal setting and goal attainment monitoring help provide the real-life experiences of focusing on and dealing with problems within the classroom. In addition, the problems raised can often generate discussions and role plays during the group sessions. Goal setting also involves teachers more closely with the program and provides one concrete indication of progress (see Chapter 3).

Preplanning

Design a Goal Sheet, similar to the model provided, that will be practical and workable in your school setting (see Appendix D). Simplicity is helpful, and having teachers initial the sheet only once during the day is usually most feasible. Collaborate with each teacher who will be monitoring goals to explain the goal-setting and monitoring process, to explain how the Goal Sheet is to be filled out, and to ask for suggestions as to the goals the teachers would like the student to be working on. It is very important to convey an openness to the teachers' input and to make the goal-setting procedures as convenient for them as possible. Make it clear that the child is responsible for the Goal Sheet and for asking the teacher to initial it; the teacher is not responsible for remembering this. Some veteran teachers, wary of the forgetfulness of children and eager to collaborate, may want to infuse more structure to ensure a successful experience. This is perfectly acceptable if it is what the teacher desires.

Because the Goal Sheets are one of the principal vehicles for generalization, care must be taken to ensure that group members understand the process. Leaders should not assume that each child understands what a "goal" is nor that the child understands why altering his or her preferred behavior to meet a goal is desirable. Modeling goal setting and attainment from the leaders' own lives is a useful training procedure. Modeling should include failure and coping with the failure through adjusting the goal. Differentiate a child's "dream" (e.g., to play in the NBA) from "goals," which are the short-term objectives that may lead toward the dream. Leaders can model their own "dreams" that were never attained and explain why, in terms of their personal willingness to accomplish necessary goals.

Note. It is common in the first two or three group meetings for the children to test the structure to see where the boundaries are. Many a new therapist has been frustrated with this behavior. Our experience has been that if the leaders adhere to the points and strikes system assiduously, reinforcing positive behavior and calling strikes on negative behavior, the vast majority of children will adjust their behavior accordingly.

Send home the first Parent Letter following this session (see Appendices I and J).

Materials

Goal Sheet and Parent Letter

Session Content

Objective 1. Review and Introduce the Concept of Setting and Realizing Goals

Review the group purpose, structure, and activities related to similarities and differences in perception. Have each group member recall one point from the previous session. Use reminders if needed.

A. Define *goal.* Most children understand it as something you work to get or do, or something you want and are willing to work for.

B. Review the overall goal of the group program: to learn the smartest way to solve problems with other people and to improve anger coping.

C. Present the Goal Sheet and explain that as part of the group program, each member will be working on a goal each week in his or her classroom that has to do with anger coping or self-control.

D. Have each group member identify a classroom problem that he or she wants to work on during the coming week. To minimize subjective judgments, help the members describe their goals in terms of observable behavior. For example, "being good in class" is very subjective, but could be behaviorally defined in terms of "not talking back to the teacher," "no physical contact with other kids," and so forth. Use information obtained from classroom teachers to indirectly influence the child's choice of goal (e.g., "How about something related to your behavior in art class?"). Strictly avoid simply prescribing the goal; clinically draw it out so that the child owns it. If the child's desired goal is unrelated to teacher concerns but reasonable, let the child go with it. There will be other opportunities.

E. Group members "vote" to decide whether all the chosen goals are roughly equivalent in terms of difficulty. It is important to select a goal that is relevant, but not so difficult as to preclude success. Have each group member write his or her goal for the week on the Goal Sheet.

F. Decide on the level of performance needed to reach the goal. Three out of 5 days is generally a good level to begin with, allowing for some lapses in behavior without ruining the entire week. Have the group members enter their required level of performance on the Goal Sheet and enter the date for the week.

G. Discuss the rules for the goal-setting procedure. The Goal Sheet is the group member's responsibility. He or she must keep track of it, make sure the teacher fills it out and signs it, and bring it back to group. No excuses are good enough for the Goal Sheet to "count" unless the rules are followed.

H. Explain the consequences of meeting a goal. Group members can earn a point to apply to the already specified group reward system. Another idea that often enlists peer pressure as a motivator is to offer a group reward, such as 5 or 10 minutes of a fun activity if everyone in the group meets his or her goal for that week. The combination of individual and group rewards provides the greatest incentive.

I. Consult with the classroom teacher when difficulties arise concerning the goal activity. The teacher may be able to provide additional guidance as to the most appropriate goals and/or the smoothest procedure for obtaining signatures.

Positive Feedback and Optional Free Time

Leaders: Debrief and Complete Case Notes

◆

SESSION 3. ANGER MANAGEMENT: PUPPET SELF-CONTROL TASK

Group Leaders' Notes

The main task in this session is to introduce the idea of thinking processes as helping to control feelings, such as anger. Children with undercontrolled or externalizing behavior problems such as aggression often suffer from *cognitive deficiencies*—lack of useful, mediating cognitions to regulate anger and the subsequent behavior (see Chapter 2). In this session the group members are introduced to the concept of adding self-talk at the appropriate time to help them to control their anger and behavior.

The skill is introduced in an indirect fashion, through the use of puppets. It is the puppet, not the child, who will be "thinking" to control its feelings while the other puppets tease and provoke it. Using this procedure is less threatening to some children and serves as a useful lead-in to Session 4, wherein the members will confront one another directly.

Leaders should obtain a puppet for each child ahead of time. (The kindergarten room is a good place to find puppets; animal or humanlike characters will do.) Leaders can also make puppets out of old sweat socks, varying their looks to the extent possible. Using valuable group time to allow the children to make their own puppets is not recommended; the taunts can easily move to the quality of the workmanship, a criticism that is too direct for this activity.

Create a circle or square "safety zone" with tape on the floor ahead of time. The child with the puppet who will be teased will stand inside the zone, so it should be made large enough that puppet-to-puppet physical contact is not possible. Six to 8 feet across is adequate.

It is advisable to help the children come up with the self-talk they will use to keep their puppet under control, well before they have their turns in the safety zone. Leader modeling will assist in this effort. Avoid allowing the activity to become a game of "tit for tat" (e.g., "Oh yeah? Well, you're uglier than I am!"). The puppet in the middle is learning to use self-control language, not one-up-manship. In addition, because those who will tease *must refrain from using swear words or racial slurs,* they may need some "thinking time" to come up with appropriate taunts.

Repeat this exercise as often as necessary until the group members appear to have a good understanding of the concept. It is typical for this session to occupy more than one meeting time.

Send home the second Parent Letter following this session.

Materials

Hand puppets, one for each group member, and Parent Letter

Session Content

Objective 1. Review Last Session and Goals

Review each child's goals from the previous week; ask the child how many days were signed. If children have done particularly well, ask them to relate what they did that helped them to reach their goals on so many days.

Objective 2. Assess Group Problem-Solving Skills

A. In a central location, place one too few puppets for each group member to have one and then instruct everyone to get a puppet for the next activity.

   Observe the problem-solving method the group uses, if any.

B. Ask the group to state the problem and discuss how they tried to solve it, what other ways could have been used to solve it, how well this way worked, and whether any rules were broken.

Objective 3. Introduce Self-Talk and Other Anger Management Techniques

Introduce the concept of self-talk, distraction techniques, and relaxation methods as affecting feelings and reactions.

A. Have one of the leaders take a puppet and receive taunts, modeling self-talk that enhances anger coping, such as "I can tell I'm starting to get mad, and I want to be careful not to get too angry and lose my temper. I think I'll ask them to stop and see if that works." Or, another possibility: "I don't want to let them make me angry and lose my temper, because then I might do something I'd be sorry for." As additional anger coping methods, model ways to *distract* your attention from the provocation (e.g., focusing on a specific visual stimulus, thinking about something fun that is planned for later in the day) and how to count to 10 while breathing deeply (or other simple relaxation methods).
B. Have each member select a puppet for the self-control game. The rule for the game is that taunts are directed at the puppets, not at group members. In addition, no racial slurs or swear words are allowed. Each puppet takes a turn receiving and responding to taunts from the rest of the group. The taunting should go on for only 20 to 30 seconds, and ample space should be kept between members to discourage physical provocation.
C. After each member's puppet receives taunts, the leaders should have the child discuss how the puppet felt, what the puppet was thinking or saying to itself, and whether the puppet used anger coping or self-control in its responses.
D. Repeat the activity, with each group member's puppet again receiving taunts and trying to use anger coping. After each member's turn, emphasize what the puppet said to itself that helped in keeping self-control.

Note. Group leaders may request that the puppets use audible vocal (or overt) self-instruction for the first go-around, moving to silent (or covert) self-instruction in subsequent turns.

Positive Feedback and Optional Free Time

Leaders: Debrief and Complete Case Notes

◆

SESSION 4. USING SELF-INSTRUCTION

Group Leaders' Notes

This session builds on the self-instruction skills introduced with the puppets in Session 3. If the leaders believe that the group members have started to grasp the concept of self-instruction to mediate anger arousal, and they can both demonstrate with puppets and verbalize the concept, then they are ready for the next level of training. At this point the puppets are put away, and the taunts are aimed by the group directly at each designated child.

It is important that the group leaders have a secure understanding of the purpose of this training procedure. Recall from Chapter 2 that angry, aggressive children often have a very limited repertoire of responses to provocative situations and that their problem-solving skills become much less competent when they simply respond "automatically" rather than use a more deliberate style. If a child has had few or no experiences with the use of deliberating to seek a more adaptive response prior to acting, chances are he or she will simply continue to execute the same aggressive response—it is what the child knows how to do. Further, a child cannot use a deliberative problem-solving style if the level of anger arousal is prohibitive to any responses other than fight or flight.

Many efforts to help children control aggressive behavior fail because the interventions do not allow for even *in vitro* experiences with the skill. Simply explaining to the children what the skills are and letting them parrot back their understanding is destined for failure. This anger coping training procedure is an attempt to create a provocative situation, within the safety of the group room, that calls on the child to actually practice anger control. In other words, we want the child to experience an anger-arousing situation, and then to actively prevent his or her anger from running its typical course. For many chronically aggressive children, this may be a first-time experience.

In this session, the children will try to provoke one another to anger, and they will try to use self-instruction to maintain anger control. We have found it respectful to ask each child if there are sensitive provocations that he or she may not be ready to handle and to abide by those wishes. However, if a particular taunt commonly triggers a child's angry outburst, that child will need to confront it at some point in the training.

Note. Just as the three most important words in real estate are "Location, location, location," the three most important words in behavioral change are "Practice, practice, practice!" The more and varied the opportunities to practice the skill, the greater the chances for generalization. Leaders should provide multiple opportunities for each child and, if possible, practice in multiple settings (e.g., the hallway, the rest room, the playground).

Materials

Deck of playing cards and dominoes, paper and pencil, a ball for pass-the-ball

Session Content

This session again emphasizes the concept of self-talk and its role in improving anger control, using activities that approximate attention to classroom tasks.

Objective 1. Review Concepts of Anger Coping or Self-Control and Goals

Review each child's goals from the previous week; ask the child how many days were signed. If some of the children have done particularly well, ask them to relate what they did that helped them to reach their goals on so many days.

Recall the self-control game from the previous session, what self-talk the group members and the leaders used, and how that helped or hurt their anger coping. If the some of members are still struggling with the idea, the concept of self-talk can be explained as being a way we talk silently to ourselves and how we figure things out. Some children have had more experience using self-talk to mediate fear, and leaders can make that connection to mediating anger. Recall who was the most successful with anger coping in the puppet exercise and how he or she did it. Encourage members to relate the taunting game to real-life experiences they encounter: "Does anyone ever try to make you angry by teasing you? What usually happens?"

Objective 2. Practice Using Anger Coping or Self-Control

A. Play a self-control memory game using playing cards. The leader picks 10 different number cards and arranges them as a fan so that all card numbers are visible. Before showing them to the selected group member, allow the other members to taunt and tease him or her for 15 seconds. *The same rules involving no racial slurs or swearing obtain here.* Then expose the cards to the selected group member for 5 seconds while the other members continue to issue verbal taunts. The one trying to remember the numbers may talk aloud. That member then writes on a separate sheet of paper as many card numbers (ignoring suits) as he or she can recall. Repeat for each group member, keeping track of how many numbers each recalls. The one with the most correct numbers wins. Be sure to keep sufficient physical distance between members.

B. Discussion: Was it hard to concentrate on the numbers? How did you keep your attention focused? Did you start to feel angry? Did that hurt your concentration? To the winner: Did you talk to yourself to help you win? Did you get angry?

C. Play a self-control game using dominoes. One group member builds a tower or constructs a line *using one hand* for 30 seconds while the others taunt. Each member takes a turn, with the highest tower or longest line winning.

D. Discuss this activity in a similar manner. Emphasize self-talk that helped and model if necessary.

E. Play the self-control game with taunts directed at group members in turn. *Leaders should model first,* uttering anger-coping "stay cool" self-statements while the group members taunt. Be sure to keep a safe distance between members. Use the same safety zone as in the previous session. The taunted one stays in the middle and responds, using anger-coping self-statements.

F. Discussion: How did you feel? What bothered you most? What were you thinking or saying to yourself? How did you use self-control?

Note. During this session, the leaders should model "stay cool" types of self-statements whenever deemed appropriate. In addition, the group members may actually need some help in coming up with taunts that are within the rules—no swear words or racial slurs. Some may find it helpful to write them down on a sheet of paper for reference. For children who have difficulty with this exercise, leaders may want to vary the verbal taunting exercises by (1) having the targeted child face away from the taunters, (2) reducing the taunting time, or (3) allowing only one or two members to taunt.

   Important. The need for "cool down" time prior to returning to class may be particularly critical following this session. A pass-the-ball exercise in which each group member states something he or she likes about another member can be useful. Relaxation exercises, such as deep breathing or pleasant imagery, are highly recommended.

Positive Feedback and Optional Free Time

Leaders: Debrief and Complete Case Notes

◆

SESSION 5. PERSPECTIVE TAKING

Group Leaders' Notes

The main idea in this session is to help group members understand that situations can be seen from different points of view, all of which have some validity. In addition, it will be important for group members to understand that a person's view may lead him or her to certain thoughts and feelings.

   This is the first "required" role play, and it is common for some of the group members to be hesitant or feel awkward. Modeling, social praise, and the awarding of points for participation can be effective motivators to get them involved.

   Note. Those leaders who will be offering point exchanges for reinforcers every fifth session should prepare for this activity. There will be no further reminders of this procedure.

Materials

Second Step (Committee for Children, 2001) or DUSO (American Guidance Service, 2001) type or other stimulus picture

Session Content

Objective 1. Review Anger Coping Skills from Last Session and Review Goals

Review each child's goals from the previous week; ask the child how many days were signed. If some of the children have done particularly well, ask them to relate what they did that helped them to reach their goals on so many days.

Ask group members whether they used their anger coping or self-control skills practiced last session. Where? How did the skills work? What might have happened if you did not use your skills?

Objective 2. Establish the Concept of Different Interpretations

A. Use a stimulus picture, such as shown on one of the DUSO or *Second Step* cards, to elicit as many perceptions of "what the problem is" as possible. Call on each group member, asking each person to come up with a different problem that *could be* happening in the picture. Repeat with other pictures if the group is interested or if it seems needed to get the point across.
B. Discuss the differences in the group members' interpretations. Was there one real problem in each picture? Would all the people in the picture see the same problem? Did you change your mind about what the problem might be in listening to the other group members' ideas? How would the people in the picture act if they all saw the same problem? If they saw different problems?

Objective 2. Problem Recognition

Help group members to recognize at what point a problem starts and reinforce the concept that each person involved in a social problem can see it differently.

A. Select a stimulus picture with a number of characters and some ambiguity, and assign a group member to portray each person in the picture. Perform a brief role play about the picture, beginning just before the scene in the picture; that is, with what led up to it. A leader assumes the role of a roving reporter and has the group freeze their action after the problem has occurred but before it is resolved. Interview each actor individually to get his or her point of view: What were you doing before the problem started? When did you first see a problem? Who had the problem? What were you thinking as the problem happened? How did you feel? What did you do? What were you planning to do next?

B. Have the group resume seats for a brief discussion. Did the people in the role play see things differently? Did they have different thoughts? Did they have different feelings? What caused those differences? Did their thoughts and feelings have an effect on what they were going to do next?

C. Ask the group members to summarize the main idea from the day's activities. Preview the next session of more role play and encourage them to bring in some real-life problems they have had, or saw others having, to use in a role play.

Positive Feedback and Optional Free Time

Leaders: Debrief and Complete Case Notes

♦

SESSION 6. LOOKING AT ANGER

Group Leaders' Notes

This session is a continuation and elaboration of the previous session, reinforcing the idea of perspective taking. It also begins to focus on the role of anger in social problems. A self-monitoring procedure is introduced.

Group leaders will now attempt to help the group members understand the feeling of anger through role play and discussion. It is likely that one or more of the group members has been involved recently in an angry episode. Such incidents make excellent role plays in the effort to help the children gain a better understanding of the feeling of anger. It is important to have the children also play the roles of others in an incident (teacher, peer provocateur, etc.) so as to help them understand the concept of seeing things from another's perspective.

Group leaders may also to choose to manufacture role plays around common school themes such as the following: A teacher blames you for something you did not do; someone accidentally rips your paper in class; someone cuts in front of you in line; someone takes your ball when you are playing. A useful insight to provide the children is that the perspective from the point of view of a peer provocateur is often, "I have the power to make _____ angry and get him (or her) in trouble." Using anger-coping strategies helps to prevent that trouble from happening.

Materials

Stimulus picture, poster paper and markers, and Hassle Logs

Session Content

Objective 1: Review Goals and Perspective Taking

Review each child's goals from the previous week; ask the child how many days were signed. If some of the children have done particularly well, ask them to relate what they did that helped them to reach their goals on so many days.

Review the concept of perspective taking, recalling last session's role-play activity.

Objective 2. Explore Situational Interpretations and Anger

Elaborate on the possibility for differing interpretations of a situation, focusing on how anger becomes involved.

A. Use a stimulus picture, or ask the group members whether they have had or have observed a problem situation that they want the group to role-play. Repeat the role-play procedure, including the roving reporter, as outlined in the previous session.
B. Using the same picture or problem situation, have the group members exchange roles and then repeat the role play.
C. Discussion: Which characters in the situation were angry? How could you tell they were angry? Was there anything about their facial expressions, their tones of voice, how they held their bodies, what they said, or what they did that showed that they were angry?
D. Repeat the role play, asking for "Academy Award winning" por-

trayals of anger by the characters who were angry, including non-verbal as well as verbal indications of anger.

E. Discuss the concept of anger. Have the group list descriptors in trying to arrive at a definition, and write these on a board or poster paper. *Suggest the idea of anger being the feeling you have when you think you cannot get something you want, or do something you want to do, or when you feel provoked.*

F. Elicit from the group examples of situations in which the children feel angry at school. Try to have the group figure out what the angry person is thinking he or she can't get or do. Talk about how the anger is a problem in itself. Generate examples of how anger gets involved in situations and how it affects what the person then chooses to do.

G. Introduce a self-monitoring, as presented in the Hassle Log (use the model shown in Appendix H or create your own.) Group members should be encouraged to examine their incidents of anger following this simple format. Hassle Logs may be filled out in subsequent meetings and used as the bases for role plays.

Positive Feedback and Optional Free Time

Leaders: Debrief and Complete Case Notes

◆

SESSION 7. WHAT DOES ANGER FEEL LIKE?

Group Leaders' Notes

The physiological aspects of anger are identified in this session, with emphasis on how they can serve as a warning sign or indicator that the person is angry and needs to mobilize anger-coping strategies. The impact of thoughts or self-statements on angry feelings and behavior is also explored.

In this session, leaders will ask the children to get in touch with the physiological sensations that accompany anger. Most adults can "sense" when they are getting angry by monitoring their physiological responses (e.g., accelerated heartbeat or breathing, muscle tension, involuntary clenching of the jaw, etc.). The "early warning system" serves as a cue for the individual to begin to cognitively deliberate the most adaptive response. It is the capacity to recognize and monitor these bodily responses, so that they may serve as a cue for the child's anger control, that will be taught in this session.

This is a difficult concept for young children, especially males, to master, unaccustomed as they often are to monitoring their feeling states. Nonetheless, it remains an important component in the effort at anger control. One must be aware that he or she is becoming angry before a decision to control that anger can be made. Abundant group leader examples and modeling help in this training (e.g., "A fellow cut me off on the highway this morning, and I could feel my teeth clench and my heart start to race"). In addition, the children may be more familiar with physiological sensations that accompany fear, which may provide a training link.

Session Content

Objective 1. Review Goals and Concepts of Anger from Last Session

Review each child's goals from the previous week; ask the child how many days were signed. If some of the children have done particularly well, ask them to relate what they did that helped them to reach their goals on so many days.

Recall the definition of anger and the examples used in the last session.

Objective 2. Identify Physiological Reactions to Anger

Explore the physiological aspects of anger arousal and how these can serve as warning signals that a problem is starting.

A. Discussion: How can we tell when we're feeling angry? How does your body feel when you are getting angry? What do you notice when others are getting angry that tells you how they might be feeling?
B. Optional: View a videotape that portrays the physiological aspects of anger arousal (see Chapter 5).
C. Discussion: People have different kinds of bodily reactions when they're having strong feelings. Have each group member describe his or her bodily changes when he or she is getting angry. Do these

bodily changes create any problems or lead to any particular behaviors? Can these bodily changes be signals that you're angry
and that there is a problem to be solved?

Objective 3. Explore Self-Statements

Explore the role of self-statements in coping with anger and redirect-
ing behavior in a problem-solving manner.

A. Discussion: What thoughts usually go along with angry feelings?
   What do you say to yourself when you're angry? Do these
   thoughts make you get angrier or stay angry? Do they help you
   calm down and try to solve the problem?
B. Optional: View a videotape that portrays two different types of
   self-statements (see Chapter 5). After the first set of angry self-
   statements, discuss whether the group members say these kinds of
   things to themselves when they're angry. Do these self-statements
   help them control their anger or solve the problem? View the second set of self-statements. Discuss whether the group members
   agreed with these thoughts. Did these self-statements help the boy
   solve his problem, help him cope with his anger?

   Have the group members specifically identify the problem the
   child had and tell what the child's feelings were, what choices the
   child had to solve the problem, and how what he said to himself
   helped him make choices.
C. Discuss incidents during the past week when someone got angry
   at school. Use the Hassle Log (see Appendix H) to guide the discussion. What did the child say to him- or herself, or what
   thoughts did he or she have? Did the thoughts or self-statements
   help with anger control? Were there things the child could have
   said to him- or herself that would have helped with anger control?
   Can self-statements help with anger control at school? Is there any
   way to remember to use them? Can the body's warning signs help
   you remember?

Positive Feedback and Optional Free Time

Leaders: Debrief and Complete Case Notes

◆

SESSION 8. CHOICES AND CONSEQUENCES

Group Leaders' Notes

The concepts presented in this session are in some ways, the most important components of the Anger Coping model in terms of helping to make changes in behavior. It is essential that group members conceive of being angry as a problem with which they need to cope, that they have different choices of things they can do when they're angry, and that there are fairly predictable consequences for their behavior.

Recall from Chapter 2 that one of the common cognitive characteristics of highly aggressive children is their deficiency in problem solving. Aggressive children demonstrate deficiency in both the quality and the quantity of their problem-solving solutions (Lochman et al., 1991). These differences are most pronounced in the quality of the solutions offered, with aggressive children offering fewer verbal assertion solutions (Asarnow & Callan, 1985; Joffe et al., 1990; Lochman & Lampron, 1986), fewer compromise solutions (Lochman & Dodge, 1994), more direct action solutions (Lochman & Lampron, 1986), a greater number of help-seeking or adult intervention responses (Asher & Renshaw, 1981; Dodge et al., 1984; Lochman, Lampron, & Rabiner, 1989; Rabiner et al., 1990), and more physically aggressive responses (Pepler et al., 1998; Slaby & Guerra, 1988; Waas, 1988; Waas & French, 1989) to hypothetical vignettes describing interpersonal conflicts.

In this session, leaders will begin to help the group members address these problem-solving deficiencies through activities that encourage them to generate multiple "choices" to previous problem incidences. The group will then review each choice and connect it to the most likely consequences that would ensue.

Note. This session is very didactic and can be too abstract for some children. Having the group members participate in an active a way is helpful in maintaining their attention. For example, let the group members take turns writing the choices or consequences they come up with on the board, writing the rankings, and so on. Be sure to give points for good participation and abundant verbal praise.

Materials

Hassle Logs, poster paper and markers

Session Content

Objective 1. Review Goals and Physiological Reactions

Review each child's goals from the previous week; ask the child how many days were signed. If some of the children have done particularly well, ask them to relate what they did that helped them to reach their goals on so many days. Review the physiological aspects of anger and the self-statements associated with anger discussed during the previous session.

Objective 2. Generate Alternatives

Encourage the process of generating alternatives, including all possible alternatives.

A. Using the Hassle Log as a guide, have the group members bring up problems that occurred during the previous week, or that they can recall from some previous time, that aroused anger. Taking one problem at a time, have the group brainstorm all the possible choices the person could have made. Emphasize the idea of *all possible choices*; leaders should offer desirable or undesirable alternatives if the group members' ideas are skewed in one direction of another. It is generally helpful to list the alternatives generated on a chalkboard or poster paper, headed by the title "Choices" or "Alternatives."

B. Once the list has been generated, go back to each choice listed and have the group decide whether the choice involved anger coping or self-control. Were there any self-statements that led to the choices? What were they? How did they affect the choices made?

Objective 3. Identify Consequences

Establish the idea of consequences as what happens after a choice is made—what others do and what happens to you—and as something to be considered in deciding on a choice.

A. Discussion: What is a consequence? This term is sometimes too sophisticated for the children, and they can more easily refer to the idea of *what happens as a result of something you do*. It can be positive or negative. Are consequences important to us? Are they one of the reasons we want to learn anger control?

B. Consider one of the problem situations discussed in Objective 2 and look again at all the choices listed. Go through the list again and predict, for each choice, the consequence, or what would happen, if that choice was made. Again, it is helpful to list the predicted consequences in another column to the right of "Choices," under the heading "What Happens."

C. Have the group rate each consequence as good or bad. Did the good consequence(s) involve anger coping or self-control? Who decides what consequence will happen? Who decides what choice is made? How are self-statements or thoughts involved in making choices and considering consequences? Can they help you make choices that lead to good consequences?

Positive Feedback and Optional Free Time

Leaders: Debrief and Complete Case Notes

◆

SESSION 9. STEPS FOR PROBLEM SOLVING

Group Leaders' Notes

The problem-solving model is presented in its entirety in this session, helping the group members to understand the sequence as an integrated process. It is important for the members to grasp the idea that this model deals with *how to think about problems*, not what to do. What happens—the content and context of problems—varies from situation to situation, but the process of how to think about problems remains the same.

Group members have learned to recognize the existence of a "problem" by considering that there may be both good and bad consequences following the possible choices. For example, they have learned that if their anger is provoked on the playground, response choices can include: (1) aggression, with possible school administrative consequences; (2) nonaggression, with possible negative peer consequences; or (3) a third choice that may avoid both types of negative consequences. Explain that the existence of these tough choices is one type of *problem*.

In this session, the group members are provided with a step model, a "cognitive map" to assist them in selecting and implementing the best choice. This session addresses the knowledge-level aspect of building applied problem-solving skills, so multiple repetitions and examples with numerous situations and contexts will assist the group members in learning the steps.

Send home the third Parent Letter following this session.

Materials

Poster paper and markers, Parent Letter

Session Content

Objective 1. Review Goals and Problem Solving

Review each child's goals from the previous week; ask the child how many days were signed. If some of the children have done particularly well, ask them to relate what they did that helped them to reach their goals on so many days. Review the steps of social problem solving, beginning with determining that there is a problem and proceeding through consideration of consequences.

A. Ask the members to recall the ideas discussed last session, prompting if necessary. On a piece of poster paper, write the steps in words the members can understand and use for themselves spontaneously. An example of steps might be as follows: (1) What is the problem?; (2) What are my feelings?; (3) What are my choices?; (4) What will happen?; (5) What will I do? A flowchart format can be used. Discuss and ask for examples of each step.

B. Ask for examples of problems the group members had during the week, and go through the steps identified. Group members should be able to relate the steps in sequence and provide an appropriate example before moving to the next objectives in Session 10.

Positive Feedback and Optional Free Time

Leaders: Debrief and Complete Case Notes

◆

SESSION 10. PROBLEM SOLVING IN ACTION

Group Leaders' Notes

This session begins the portion of the training wherein the group members take a more active role in rehearsing the skills to address their own particular anger-related needs. Over the course of the remaining weeks, the children will create, rehearse, and videotape one or more vignettes that depict the skills they are learning. It is important that the problems that are created by the group members reflect actual and recurring difficulties that they encounter in the school setting. This session prepares the group members for this task by presenting a common problem and discussing alternative responses.

Session 10 assumes that the leaders have prepared an example videotape ahead of time or have a copy of *The Anger Coping Video*, available from either of us. (See Chapter 5 for guidelines.) An effective example video can be made very simply before the start of this group session. Position a volunteer child who is the same age or slightly older than the group members at a desk with the camera just on him or her, so that the child takes up most of the frame. The child ("Terry") should be writing in a workbook or on a piece of writing paper, obviously engaged in the assignment, not talking. Off camera an adult voice says, "That's enough talking back there. Terry that was your last warning. You go to the principal's office right now!" With that same setup, tape three different responses to the problem: (1) poor anger control, disrespectful; (2) passive, unassertive; and (3) good anger control, assertive, and respectful. Alternately, this session may be completed by having the group members role-play with the leader. The critical feature is analysis of the alternative responses.

Materials

Prepared videotape

Session Content

Objective 1. Review Goals and Present the Problem-Solving Model in Action

Review each child's goals from the previous week; ask the child how many days were signed. If some of the children have done particularly well, ask them to relate what they did that helped them to reach their goals on so many days.

A. Explain to the group that they will be making a videotape themselves during the next 6 weeks, which will show how anger coping works. Point out that you have a model for them to watch that will give them an idea of what they will be trying to do.
B. View a videotape in which a boy is blamed by the teacher for something he didn't do. It will be important to stop the videotape between each alternative solution that is acted out, to help the members understand that after each pause the scene returns to the point when the boy is angry and deciding what choice to make.
C. After the *first alternative* is shown, stop the videotape for discussion. What is the problem? When did it start? Whose problem is it? How is the boy feeling? How can he tell, and how can you tell, that he is angry? What angry thoughts might he be having? What could he be telling himself? What choice did he make? What was the consequence? Did he make a smart choice?
D. After the *second alternative* is shown, stop for discussion. Did the boy have the same problem? Did he have the same feelings? What choice did he make? (called the teacher a name; gave up; failed to be assertive). What happened? Did he make a smart choice?
E. After the *third alternative*, discuss the tape. What were the three choices on the tape? Which one was the smartest choice? Which choices used anger control? What did the boy say to himself that helped him use anger control? (Emphasize a motto such as "Stop, think, what should I do?") Can the children think of any other choices? What would happen as a result of those choices?
F. Remind the group that at the next meeting they will begin working on a script for the videotape they will make. Encourage group members to come up with ideas for their videotape.

Positive Feedback and Optional Free Time

Leaders: Debrief and Complete Case Notes

◆

SESSION 11. VIDEO PRODUCTION I

Group Leaders' Notes

This session marks the beginning of the actual effort to produce a video that demonstrates what is being learned in the Anger Coping group. This process helps to consolidate the integrated problem-solving model begun in Session 9. By writing their own script, the group begins to acquire a working knowledge of the social problem-solving process. Another important goal for this session is to defuse some of the anxiety and impulse-control problems generally elicited by the videotaping process.

Our experience with this phase of the training causes us to advise the following:

1. Group leaders should become proficient with the video technology ahead of time and be certain that it is in working order.
2. Leaders should resist group members' desire to rush to on-camera production. Be satisfied that they have rehearsed sufficiently so that the vignette is "camera-ready" before beginning to tape. Be prepared for multiple "takes," however.
3. Moving the setting to the actual locale (e.g., the gym or outside on the playground) and including other salient individuals such as a teacher or administrator adds realism and offers potentially greater generalization possibilities.
4. Large poster-sized signs can be used to introduce scenes (e.g., "What Is the Problem?").
5. The use of written, cartoonlike "thought bubbles" on a stick held over an actor's head can portray self-instruction. Alternately, one of the off-camera group members can speak into the microphone of the video camera while the on-camera actor shows "thinking."

Materials

Poster paper and markers, Hassle Logs, and video equipment

Session Content

Objective 1. Review Goals and Identify Problems in School

Review each child's goals from the previous week; ask the child how many days were signed. If some of the children have done particularly well, ask them to relate what they did that helped them to reach their goals on so many days. Identify one of several problems in school that the group believes would be good to videotape, establishing one problem as first priority for filming.

A. Remind the group of the videotape shown during the last session. Ask for suggestions of problem situations in school involving anger arousal that group members think would be good for making a videotape.
B. Write down on a piece of paper or poster paper each problem suggested, determine whether it does involve anger, and ask for three or four choices the person with the problem might make and the consequences that would occur. Be certain to have the group include choices involving self-control, as well as at least one that does not. The Hassle Log can provide possible scenarios.
C. Once choices and consequences have been outlined for each problem, have the group decide which problem they would most like to videotape first. Explain that if the taping goes well, there will be opportunity to make more than one tape. Having the group reach this decision can prove to be a real-life demonstration of problem solving. Point this out and see what choices the group can find as a whole.

Objective 2. Desensitize the Group to Being on Camera

Give each group member a chance to be on camera informally, allowing the laughter and silliness that invariably occur. It will still be necessary for members to retain some degree of self-control. In addition, it can be fun to practice some close-up shots, with the group members asked to portray different emotions. At the end of the session, play the tape back so that the group members can watch themselves. It is also important to establish a policy about handling the equipment to prevent damage.

Positive Feedback and Optional Free Time

Leaders: Debrief and Complete Case Notes

◆

SESSION 12–18. VIDEO PRODUCTIONS II–VIII

Group Leaders' Notes

During these sessions, the group should begin to work more seriously on producing part of their videotape. Although it is important to encourage the children to do their best job of acting so as to make a good product, leaders should continue to keep in mind that this taping activity is primarily a *training* activity. The goal is to help the children internalize the problem-solving model, and the video project is the vehicle to help reach that goal. Our experience—and that of many of our students—is that it is easy to become swept away into the novelty and technology of video production and lose sight of that primary goal. Consequently, it is advisable for leaders to remain particularly observant of the developing skill levels of each of the group members as rehearsals progress, and to develop refined training objectives prior to each upcoming session.

Materials

Video equipment, paper and pencil

Session 12 Content: Video Production II

Objective 1. Review Goals and Tape the Problem Situation

Review each child's goals from the previous week; ask the child how many days were signed. If some of the children have done particularly well, ask them to relate what they did that helped them to reach their goals on so many days. Tape a clear representation of the problem stem, which leads into an initially inappropriate, angry/aggressive action that has negative consequences for the individual.

A. Review the problem decided upon by the group. Lay out the scene and the circumstances that lead up to the problem. Assign roles (which can be another group problem-solving process) and arrange scenery. Decide on the actions and words used by each character, writing them down if necessary (although it usually is not).

B. Have several "dress rehearsals" of role plays of the problem. Begin with setting the stage, what leads up to the problem, then have the problem occur, and stop when the person with the problem is looking very angry. (One of these taped rehearsals may be good enough for a final version.) The group will continue to do these "dress rehearsals" for subsequent segments of the videotape as well.
C. Allow the group to watch the replays of their videotaped rehearsals, keeping these questions in mind: Is the problem presented clearly? Can the actors be understood? Is there too much extraneous noise of silliness? How is the anger displayed? Did the important action of the sequence get on camera? Would someone from outside the group understand the problem from watching the tape? After watching the replay, decide what changes need to be made on the next taping, giving specific suggestions.
D. An additional feature that may be added to the problem stem is a roving reporter or narrator who interviews the actors while the action is frozen, as in the role-play activities for Session 5. Get a close-up of the person being interviewed, having him or her respond as an aside to the audience, telling what he is thinking, feeling, and so on.
E. Select and tape a solution choice that demonstrates lack of anger control.

Positive Feedback and Optional Free Time

Leaders: Debrief and Complete Case Notes

Session 13 Content: Video Production III

This session continues the videotaping efforts, moving to the various alternatives and consequences in the script.

Objective 1. Review Goals and Prepare for Taping of Alternatives and Consequences

Review each child's goals from the previous week; ask the child how many days were signed. If some of the children have done particularly well, ask them to relate what they did that helped them to reach their goals on so many days.

A. Watch the group's videotape of the problem stem and angry/aggressive solution that was selected as the final version.
B. Prepare any props that the group decides to include in their tape, such as signs saying "Stop, think, what should I do?" or listing the steps in the problem-solving process the group has outlined.

Objective 2. Tape the Alternative Solutions

Videotape a clear representation of each alternative and associated consequence, using only alternatives that involve self-control of anger arousal.

Positive Feedback and Optional Free Time

Leaders: Debrief and Complete Case Notes

Sessions 14–18 Content: Video Productions IV–VIII

These sessions review the group's videotape product and the concepts presented during the group's meetings and apply the concepts to the group members' anger arousal problems. Leaders should continue with the goal reviews through the conclusion of the intervention.

Objective 1

View the "finished products," giving comments about strengths and weaknesses.

Objective 2 (Optional)

Produce videotapes of other problem stems, alternatives, and consequences. These problems can focus on different types of anger arousal problems, such as with adults rather than with peers.

Objective 3

Review the steps of social problem solving, giving group members an opportunity to offer what they recall before the leaders fill in.

Objective 4

Review the progress group members have made in anger coping, asking for many specific examples of situations in which group members have used their skills. Reference to the Goal Sheets may be helpful.

Objective 5

Preview how group members anticipate being able to use their newly acquired anger-coping skills in the future.

Objective 6

Train for the eventuality of setbacks, such as how to cope with possible situations in which the newly acquired skills may be neglected in favor of aggression. Remind the group members that they are learning to "cope" with anger, not "master" it, and sometimes they will not be successful. Remind them that they don't quit a basketball game after a missed shot or a bad pass. Rather, they try to learn from the error and continue playing. Coping with anger and aggression requires the same kind of commitment to learning from errors and moving on. Coping with setbacks may include:

> *Self-coaching*: "What did I forget to do?" "How can I handle this better next time?" "What step did I forget?" "I know how to do it, I just need practice." "One mistake doesn't spoil all the work I've done." "I'll do better next time."
>
> *Seeking help*: Ask to see one of the group leaders for an individual session to help you improve your skills.

Objective 7

Plan a "graduation" ceremony. Our experience has been that the group members appreciate a closing ritual, which may include personalized Anger Coping Program certificates (made with a word processing certificate-maker program), invited adult guests, snacks, and the opportunity to show their videotape and talk about what they have learned.

CHAPTER 8

♦♦♦

Frequently Asked Questions

♦

Q: I noticed that most of the theoretical and research foundations in Chapters 2 and 6 involved boys as subjects. Can the Anger Coping Program (ACP) be used with girls as well?

A: Literally all of the research on the ACP involved boys. This decision was made in part because boys are at considerably higher risk, as a gender, for externalizing behavior problems and the subsequent mental health and legal difficulties that may follow in the developmental trajectory. That said, there is no reason that practitioners should not use the program with girls who are demonstrating anger control problems, particularly if such problems are manifested as reactive physical aggression. In other words, the more the girls' anger resembles the boys' anger, the higher the likelihood that the ACP will be an appropriate intervention. Note, however, that there is a growing body of research that suggests that girls may experience and express anger and aggression in a somewhat different manner than boys (see Crick, 1997; Crick & Bigbee, 1998; Crick & Werner, 1998; but see also Pepler & Sedighdeilami, 1998, for additional viewpoints). In general, this literature indicates that many more girls than boys may use what is called "relational aggression." This is typically a nonphysical form of aggression that often involves using social exclusion, rumor spreading, and mean-spirited teasing as a form of retaliation. Practitioners are advised to become familiar with this literature before beginning work with girls.

Q: May I combine girls and boys in the same group?

A: This is acceptable if your assessment indicates similar anger and aggression expression patterns. As the children get older, inhibitions in regard to role playing and possible behavioral management problems associated with burgeoning sexuality may become of concern. As a rule, gender-specific groups work best.

Q: What are the upper and lower age ranges for the ACP?

A: The bulk of the existing research on the ACP has been done with boys in the 8- to 12-year-old range. Clinically, both of us have worked with children somewhat younger and somewhat older, and this can be a successful experience if the appropriate adaptations are made. For instance, with older middle school students, we have eliminated the puppet self-control activity, replacing it with additional work from the subsequent "real life" self-control activity. When working with very young children, group leaders should attend carefully to developmental variables. Younger children need to "do and see" to a greater degree than their older peers, and this has implications for the more cognitive aspects of the ACP. Sessions need to be shorter, less didactic, and contain abundant use of manipulatives and behavioral rehearsal. Young children are quite capable of developing problem-solving skills, but, again, developmental status is a major consideration. (See Shure, 1996, for a useful, research-supported guide for problem-solving work with preschool and kindergarten children.)

Q: How many children per group is an optimal number?

A: This varies, depending on a few factors, including room size and number of leaders. With two group leaders and sufficient space, five to seven children is a good target. Avoid allowing the "group" to become more like a "class" with the addition of too many children, thus increasing behavioral management problems and reducing opportunities for more individualized attention. Single group leaders will find four to five children to be sufficient. This number is large enough to account for the inevitable absences and still allow for "group-type" activities.

Q: Can we meet more than once per week?

A: Certainly, but not if the goal is to rush through the sessions to meet a school deadline or some other target date. Give yourself enough time to have the children *in treatment* at least 16 to 18 weeks. If you are planning a second-semester group, this may mean getting started with identification and parent consents before the holiday break to give yourself plenty of time.

Q: How long should each session be?

A: Forty-five minutes to an hour is a good target figure.

Q: Can I add some activities that I learned from another intervention, or must I limit myself to what is found in the ACP manual?

A: The procedures contained in the ACP manual are those that have been shown to be effective in our research. That said, we can think of no reason that the addition, rather than substitution, of other rationally conceived cognitive-behavioral activities that address the training objectives should not be included by experienced group leaders. This holds true for creative behavioral management procedures as well. Indeed, we would appreciate being informed of any useful modifications.

Q: I am uncomfortable with the teasing activity that goes on in the self-control sessions. Don't they do enough of that on their own without having to "practice" it in the counseling room?

A: The self-control sessions are specifically created to produce in each identified child a *need*, however artificial, to exert self-control, anger-coping strategies. We know of no other way, short of following the children around all day, to allow them to practice the skills needed. The self-control sessions are analogous to going out the first time in the driver's education car on the practice track: It's not the real condition, but it is close enough to stimulate the new driver's skill development. This helps ensure that the skills needed in the eventual "real thing" are practiced and thus potentially accessible under the more highly stressful conditions of the public highways. Similarly, children who lack the skills to adaptively manage anger and aggression need to spend quality time on the therapy "practice track" before they can be expected to more skillfully navigate the higher-stress conditions of the authentic school and home environments.

Q: Can I use the ACP in my clinic practice?

A: Certainly, although adaptations to achieve generalization will have to be made. In such cases, enlisting the parent/guardian—rather than the classroom teacher—as the principal collaborator for goals and other generalization activities makes sense. In a residential treatment setting, both house parents/unit counselors and school staff may be engaged for these purposes.

Q: Is there a similar program for high school students?

A: Consider the following:

Feindler, E. L., & Scalley, M. (1999). Adolescent anger-management groups for violence reduction. In T. Kratochwill & K. Stoiber (Eds.), *Handbook of group interventions for children and families* (pp. 100–119). New York: Allyn & Bacon.

Goldstein, A. P., Glick, B., & Gibbs, J. C. (1998). *Aggression replacement training: A comprehensive intervention for aggressive youth.* Champaign, IL: Research Press.

Hammond, W. R. (1991). *Dealing with anger: A violence prevention program for African-American youth.* Champaign, IL: Research Press.

Larson, J. (1994). Cognitive-behavioral treatment of anger-induced aggression in the school setting. In M. J. Furlong & D. C. Smith (Eds.), *Anger, hostility, and aggression: Assessment, prevention, and intervention strategies for youth* (pp. 393–440). Brandon, VT: Clinical Psychology. (This is a discussion of the *Think First Program.*)

Q: How do I contact the authors?

A: Jim Larson
Department of Psychology
University of Wisconsin–Whitewater
Whitewater, WI 53190
E-mail: *larsonj@mail.uww.edu*

John E. Lochman
Department of Psychology
University of Alabama
348 Gordon Palmer
Box 870348
Tuscaloosa, AL 35487-0348
E-mail: *jlochman@gp.as.ua.edu*

CHAPTER 9

◆◆◆

Case Example

◆

Jenna was a first-year school psychologist who provided services to Lincoln Elementary School, located in a medium-size, industry-based community in South Central Wisconsin. One of the first things she noticed when she arrived at the school was the seemingly high volume of children who were referred for special education services. In particular, children at Lincoln were being referred at the highest frequency to programs for pupils with emotional and behavior disabilities (EBD). In fact, the referral and placement rates were well above the state and national averages for this category of disability.

A little investigation on her part turned up a possible contributing explanation: The recently retired previous school psychologist was of the "old school," and although he was very skilled at individual assessment, he offered little else in his service delivery model. In addition, there was no functional building consultation team to support the teachers. Children with behavior problems either adjusted to the school and classroom discipline structure, or were routinely suspended or referred to special education. This model ran counter to everything that Jenna had learned in her training and was inconsistent with both the spirit and letter of the Individuals with Disabilities Education Act (IDEA). Change was in order, she thought.

Following a number of meetings with key administrative, supportive services, and teaching staff, Jenna spent much of her first year setting up the structure for a more prevention-oriented approach to service delivery (see, e.g., Minke & Bear, 2000; Ysseldyke et al., 1997). The first order of business was to get a useful building consultation team (BCT) organized, trained, and functioning (e.g., Sprick, 1999). This was a challenge, due mostly to the teachers' comfort with the traditional "test and place" model they had grown used to, but she persisted. Teachers who have been routinely "rescued" by special education are often loathe to make changes that may mean additional burdens to their already heavy responsibilities (Skrtic, 1991). Ultimately, however, increasing occurrences of effective classroom interventions through the consultation process soon began to win over many of the staff.

Jenna knew that along with indirect service delivery, an essential ingredient to an effective prevention-oriented model of service delivery was direct skill training for those children at high risk. Her university education had included training and supervised practice in the Anger Coping Program, so when an increasing number of referrals to the BCT began to include children with anger and aggression difficulties, she decided to see whether the situation warranted this form of intervention. Jenna consulted with a number of teachers and made the decision to form a group consisting of fourth-grade boys. She enlisted the support of the school guidance counselor as a co-leader.

Following the procedures she had learned in her university training, Jenna used the multiple-gate screening system (see Chapter 3) and eventually identified five fourth-grade boys for her group. With parental consents on file, she met with each of the boys individually, discussed the group, and asked them to complete the Children's Inventory of Anger (Nelson & Finch, 2000), a Likert scale measure of the affective component of anger expression to a series of trigger statements (e.g., "Someone rides your bike without permission"). She then obtained from the office records a count of discipline referrals for each child, extending back to the start of the school year. Teachers were asked to complete the Teacher Rating Scale from the Behavior Assessment System for Children (Reynolds & Kamphaus, 1992) to screen for co-occurring problems.

Satisfied that the identified children could potentially benefit from the Anger Coping Program, Jenna began the process of enlisting the teachers as full collaborators in the skills-training effort. Because there were three different teachers, she arranged to meet them all as a group one day before the start of school. At this meeting, she explained the objectives of the training, session by session, and brainstormed with the teachers how they could serve as generalization facilitators in the their classrooms. Two of the teachers were receptive to this new role, but a third still clung to her belief that her student belonged in special education and was resistant to putting forth "extra effort." Nevertheless, Jenna obtained useful information from the teachers to guide her in the goal-setting activities and scheduled times to consult with each on a weekly basis.

A week prior to the first meeting, she and her co-leader met to discuss behavior management strategies for the group. It was agreed that Jenna would be in charge of the skills training while the guidance counselor handled the points, strikes, and other necessary behavior management responsibilities. They obtained a small budget from the school fund and purchased a number of school-related items to be used as reinforcers. A donation from the parent organization allowed them to purchase snacks as well. Jenna believed that she was ready.

(The following is from an e-mail that Jenna sent to one of us [Larson] after her first group meeting.)

The first meeting was an example of worst-case scenario. I went to retrieve the five boys from their classrooms and two took off in opposite directions down the hall. The other three walked with me down to the meeting room. I asked the guidance counselor to stay with them while I went to find the other two. Fetching the other two was something of a hunting expedition. I went down to the end of one hall where I saw the two boys together and when I got there, they were gone. I walked down the stairs and down to the other end of the hall. Still no one. So, I went back up the stairs at the other end of the hall and repeated my pathway. This time, I noticed a head peeping out from behind the utility cabinet at the base of the stairs. I retrieved that child and asked the guidance counselor to contain him while I found the other boy. While I was looking for him, the guidance counselor got a phone call for which he had to go to another room to answer. In the meantime, the "lost boy" came and got his runaway buddy and off they ran.

About this time, a teacher asked what I was doing and if she could help. She suggested we look in the boys' bathroom. We did and found the two boys wetting down the Nerf ball that was a prop for our first session. After escorting them back to the group room and after the thirty-minute search, I was ready to begin session one. Such would not be the case.

One boy began punching at the walls and running around touching everything. He grabbed his buddy and then he curled up in the corner with his buddy and refused to sit in his seat. His buddy just lay there sucking his thumb and saying to me, "I have ADHD and I had sugar this morning." Then, one boy called another a name and a fist-fight broke out. In the midst of all this, there was a break-through of sorts. When I was finally able to introduce the point system, one boy said that after earning so many points, he would like to put on a show for the group. I told him that would be a great idea except that he would have to earn some points first. We began in earnest.

Things were going better until the "lost boy" who initially didn't want to come to the meeting now did not want to leave after he earned three strikes. He grabbed onto the table legs with his hands and feet and said, "No! I don't want to go. You can't make me go." The principal happened by and hearing the commotion, threatened to call the child's mother if he didn't go back to his classroom as instructed. He went. The saga continues. . . . (Jenna S., personal communication, February, 2001).

Jenna and her co-leader regrouped for the next session. They met with the most problematic boys individually and more carefully explained the group and its behavioral expectations. They also set up a "transition points" schedule to reinforce appropriate movement in and out of the classroom and practiced the behavior with the boys individually. The second meeting went much more smoothly, and they made it through the Session 1 objectives without major incident. The same boy had three strikes again, but returned uneventfully to his room. Although he continued to be something of a challenge as the training progressed, this was his last "three strikes" removal from the group.

Jenna met with each of the teachers on a weekly basis to inform them of the progress in the group and to encourage the teachers to watch for and reinforce incidences of anger control observed in the authentic setting. Teachers also provided her with information regarding the behavioral and social issues currently faced by the group members so as to help her to make her training efforts as relevant as possible. One teacher was especially adept at suggesting role plays, and another devised a system to help ensure that the Goal Sheet was signed daily and returned. Unfortunately, the teacher who started out resistant remained that way throughout the course of the intervention and used the meeting time to vent her anger about her student (and other children as well). She was a younger woman, nowhere near retirement, so Jenna decided that this relationship was an investment in possibly many children to come and dutifully kept her appointments and positive attitude. She made a mental note about working to secure classroom discipline training for the staff for next year—and possibly some stress management workshops.

As the sessions progressed, Jenna kept an ongoing record of discipline referrals for the boys in her group. She graphed them for each of the group members so she could monitor one of the outcome goals of the intervention as they progressed. Two of the teachers agreed to complete goal attainment scaling (GAS) forms for her, and she maintained those results on a line graph.

In the group, the puppet self-control sessions went very well, but once the puppets were put away in the succeeding meeting, one of the boys had a little more difficulty. During the taunting exercise, the first boy in the "safety circle" had a problem using his self-control techniques and bolted from the room. Once retrieved, he agreed to watch as the others took their turns, and they did particularly well. Jenna offered the first child another opportunity. He declined, but at the next meeting agreed to try it again with only one of the boys and Jenna doing the taunting. This was somewhat more successful. Ultimately, although the other boys achieved effective self-control with the use of self-instruction, this child decided to use the technique of leaving the scene when he felt his anger aroused.

To make an effort at enhancing generalization, at the next meeting Jenna and her co-leader took the self-control exercise out of the group room and into the natural school environment. They practiced the taunting self-control exercise on the playground, at a pickup basketball game, in the hallway, and in the lunchroom. One of the boys noted the similarity with the popular "trash talking" on the basketball court and concluded that if he could handle it there, he could handle it other places too.

"In basketball, they just trying to get you off your game, but you don't let 'em," he said. "And in school, they just trying to get you in trouble, and you don't let 'em do that either."

"I wanted to hug him!" Jenna reported. "But, instead, I stayed the good school psychologist and enthusiastically praised his insight."

The first opportunity to cash in acquired points for school merchandise came at the fifth session. Points were tallied and exchanged for tickets taken from a ticket roll obtained by the group leaders. Because the leaders had made an effort to provide points at a generally equal rate among the children (often not an easy task), everyone was enthusiastic about participating. "I will never again underestimate the value to a fourth grader of a brand new rubber eraser," Jenna reported.

When it eventually came time to make their video, the group was energized by the task. The group leaders taught the boys the "brainstorming" process: free opportunity to suggest anything, and no criticism allowed. After their normal Goal Sheet review, they spent an entire meeting brainstorming possible scenarios, with the co-leader writing them on the chalkboard as they went along. At the next meeting, they narrowed the choices to three: a pushing incident on a basketball court, a mistaken accusation of student misbehavior by a teacher, and a tripping incident in the lunchroom that may or may not have been an accident.

The group leaders decided that next task was script writing but soon discovered that the boys were considerably better at improvisation than they were at writing, so the "scripts" became only general notes about who was to be in what role in each scenario. (*Note:* It has been our experience that groups can go in either direction with script writing for the video. Some want to produce complex, dialogue-driven "masterpieces," whereas others prefer to just "wing it" until it comes out right. Our advice is to follow the lead of the group members on this issue.) Each scenario was assigned a "director" from the group, whose responsibility was to organize the cast, assign roles, and be in charge of the rehearsals. Following in the Hitchcock tradition, directors were also allowed walk-on parts in their videos. On a directive from the principal, however, the boys were not allowed to operate the school's video camera.

"By this time the boys were very attuned to the expected behaviors in the group and were virtually no management problem," Jenna reported. "Consequently, as the leaders, we had to continually remind ourselves that the video was *training*, not just a school project with a bunch of fourth graders."

If the leaders needed reminding that the boys were in need of continuing skill development, the rest of the school apparently did not. In the middle of making the video, two of the boys were suspended from school for 3 days for participating in a brawl on the school bus, and a third had an in-school suspension and parent conference for calling the art teacher "a fat hog lady" and pushing over an easel.

The video production was halted while the group addressed the particular issues surrounding the fight and the failure to maintain self-control in the art room. The Hassle Logs were used to structure the incidents and allow for self-evaluation. Role plays were then set up to recreate the events and practice anger-coping responses. The group leaders sought but were denied permission to take one of the role plays onto an actual school bus for practice, so they made do by aligning chairs bus-style in the group room.

The art teacher was remarkably forgiving and professional, and she agreed to participate in a series of role plays with both the offending child and the other group members. The art room was apparently a "trigger" environment for self-control problems of many sorts, and the teacher was eager to address them in the context of the boys' training. She was also open to suggestions from Jenna regarding classroom management strategies.

With the latest disciplinary concerns finally addressed to the satisfaction of the group leaders and the boys, they returned to producing the video. The "tripping incident in the lunchroom" scenario was replaced with the bus fight incident. This was decided upon both because of the immediate relevancy and the fact that, because of all the previous practice and repetition (in the role plays), it was now "camera ready." After five or so "takes," the group agreed on the best one and moved on to the other scenarios.

The group continued for 4 more weeks while they completed the other video vignettes, maintaining a training focus and continuing work on the classroom goals as they progressed. When all of the videos were finally "in the can," they set a date for their graduation event. It was decided that each group member could invite parents and one adult from the school. Because of the parents' work schedules, the event was scheduled for 6:00 P.M. Each boy invited his classroom teacher (unfortunately, only two accepted), and the leaders invited the principal and the art teacher.

Everyone met in the school library, feasting on cupcakes and soda while the boys explained what they had been learning and proudly showed their videos. The leaders had prepared a Certificate of Completion for each of the children and distributed the certificates with as much pomp as the situation would allow. Certificates of Appreciation were also given to parents and teachers. It was a rare and proud moment for these high-risk children and their parents.

The group leaders scheduled booster sessions and gathered the boys together at the set intervals for problem solving and role plays. Postgroup data derived from discipline reports and GAS ratings showed a positive trend, if not necessarily a statistically significant one, for four of the boys during treatment and at booster session intervals. The fifth child (whose teacher was *you know who*) continued to struggle, but primarily in the environment of classroom, not on the playground or the bus. All were subsequently promoted to the fifth grade, and none was referred for special education. Jenna and her co-leader made plans to reassemble the group at the start of school in September for additional booster sessions and ongoing support with their fifth-grade teachers.

Note: Appreciation is extended to the real "Jenna" and the many other practitioners and interns whose accumulated experiences with the Anger Coping Program are also represented in this case example.

CHAPTER 10

♦♦♦

Afterword

♦

POSTTREATMENT EVALUATION

In our many years of working in schools and with school personnel, we have heard both hard-working counselors and school psychologists evaluate their recently completed group counseling experience in words such as these:

"I think it went well."
"The kids seemed to enjoy it, and they worked hard."
"I think the teachers were pleased."
"The principal told me she was really glad somebody had worked with these kids."

Typically, these individuals could not produce any other useful outcome data, beyond this informal adult social validation, to support the efficacy of their often very considerable effort. The reasons for this lack were varied, but they generally came down to the fact that the practitioners simply failed to see the need. The mere fact that they had chosen to actually "do something" with some of the most disruptive children in the school often provided enough social approval from staff and parents to make any other form of data gathering seem unnecessary. Whether the children changed demonstrably in any positive fashion became almost irrelevant to the fact that at least the effort was made. We can speak from personal experience: Professional approval from teachers and administrators is powerful stuff for most supportive services staff.

Although the approval of peers and parents is often desirable and important, by itself it should be insufficient for the effective school practitioner. The need for data-based decision making in considering both the needs of children and the issues associated with professional accountability argue compellingly for the acquisition of more substantial data. Using research-supported interventions, such as the Anger Coping Program, is certainly the start, as it increases the likelihood that desired outcomes will be forthcoming. In addition, empirically validated interventions are more easily supportable in the face of outside scrutiny of accountability. Moving on to gather useful outcome data that speak to the relative effectiveness of the intervention is the next critical step.

Some practitioners may shy away from this form of outcome measurement, fearing a lack of knowledge in either program evaluation or research design. However, an applied evaluation of the effects of a school intervention need not be complex or rigorously designed. Face it: It isn't going to published in the *Journal of Applied Behavioral Analysis*. What the practitioner is looking for is simply data to document that the anticipated objectives were met. Did the children achieve many or most of their classroom goals as recorded on the Goal Sheets? Are the children engaging in fewer anger-related fights or disruptions as documented in classroom and office records? Does a teacher checklist (e.g., Achenbach, 1991; Dodge & Coie, 1987; Reynolds & Kamphaus, 1992), completed before the group started and then repeated at postintervention, indicate positive changes in the classroom? Do the children's postintervention self-reports indicate increased understanding of problem-solving skills or anger control in comparison with preintervention levels?

Using permanent products data acquired during the identification phase can be extremely helpful in documenting clinically useful changes (see Chapter 3). Baseline levels of discipline reports and other authentic school data acquired prior to the start of the intervention can serve as comparison points for similar data acquired during and following the intervention. Moreover, if these data are continuously monitored as the intervention proceeds, in the manner of a *formative evaluation*, adjustments and refinements can be made along the way. The practitioner is looking only for *positive trends*, not statistical significance.

Examine the convergence of multiple sources of data. Data from a single source may be unimpressive when viewed alone, but when added to data from additional sources, a converging trend may be readily observable. For instance, the teacher postintervention checklist may show very little pre- to postintervention positive gain in the targeted behaviors as measured by the externalizing scales of the BASC (Reynolds & Kamphaus, 1992). However, when these data are examined along with even modest reductions in office referrals, a majority of goals met, and an improvement in academic grades, then the converging evidence can be thought of as clinically positive.

The information gleaned from formative and summative assessments are meant to assist the practitioner in refining later iterations of the intervention, as well as to provide him or her with documentation that may be useful in subsequent school or district accountability exercises. The data may be thereafter rendered to graph form for easy dissemination to interested parties, with confidentiality maintained, of course (e.g., Child 1, Child 2, and so forth).

BOOSTER SESSIONS

It is essential to maintenance and generalization efforts that the leaders plan for additional group meetings over the rest of the school year. As with the learning and application of other psychosocial skills, children can forget, develop alternative but inappropriate habits, or simply fail to implement such skills. Booster sessions can help to reinforce and strengthen previous learning and provide the group members with an opportunity to address newly arisen issues. A suggested schedule is as follows:

Booster 1: Three weeks after the final session
Booster 2: Five weeks after the final session
Booster 3: Prior to summer

Use of the Hassle Log procedure at the booster sessions to help the children to maintain skills learned in the Anger Coping sessions is recommended. In addition, previous classroom goals should be reviewed, and the children should use their problem-solving skills to address any backsliding or newly arisen difficulties. These sessions should be informal, but group leaders should remember the caveat:

"Practice, practice, practice." Discussion is important, but insufficient: Get the group members up and role playing the current concerns. (In addition, we have found that having the group members' video ready for playing—sometimes repeatedly—is always a good idea.)

ADDITIONAL MAINTENANCE
AND GENERALIZATION

In addition to conducting booster sessions, the following are recommended to help the children maintain their skills and generalize them to authentic settings:

1. Keep in close contact with the classroom teacher(s) regarding the behavior of the group members, both during and after the intervention. Use the *Anger Coping Classroom Generalization In-service Guide* (see Appendix C) to assist the teacher. See the group members individually, as may be needed.

2. Consult with the teacher regarding classroom or recess discipline or behavior management programs. Encourage incentives that emphasize the anger-management skills trained in the group.

3. Inform administrators of the skills trained in the Anger Coping Program and encourage them to reinforce the group members when appropriate.

4. Meet with parents to help problem solve home difficulties that may have a direct impact on school behavior. Provide parent management training when possible.

5. Have recent "graduates" give talks to classes of younger students (e.g., K–3) about what they have learned, using their video as a teaching tool.

6. Encourage teachers to place graduates in appropriate positions of responsibility, such as playground monitor, so as to allow them to exercise their newly acquired skills in a prosocial manner.

7. Engage alumni from previous Anger Coping groups to serve as "consultants" to newer groups. Allow them to explain what they have learned and provide teaching models for the

younger children at selected times during the intervention. Meichenbaum and Biemiller's (1998) book, *Nurturing Independent Learners: Helping Students Take Charge of Their Learning* is an excellent resource on the subject of maintenance and generalization for a variety of learning tasks, including the use of the "consultant" role.

ONGOING NEEDS

Practitioners working with highly externalizing children are cautioned about a possible negative phenomenon that may arise. It had been our experience that some well-meaning but misguided teachers and administrators have unrealistic expectations about the effects of even well-designed anger-control interventions. Consequently, if one or more of the children do not exhibit obvious and dramatic behavioral changes following the intervention, those children may be subject to undue punitive responses—"Well, look at all the effort we made for him, and he still chooses to act this way!"

When retributive attitudes develop among adult staff members, the potential for inappropriate educational planning and behavioral consequences escalates. Negative biases toward the child can potentially result in increased use of empirically unsupported behavioral consequences such as suspensions from school, corporal punishment, and even inappropriate referral to special education.

Practitioners should remind fellow staff members that for some individuals, aggression is a very stable behavioral response, and the likelihood is high that some children who have successfully completed the entire Anger Coping Program will need continued intervention as they progress through school. If a child does well during his participation in the group but regresses to old behavioral habits in succeeding months, practitioners should help others to *take that as data, not failure*. Some children need insulin, some need psychostimulant medication, and others need hearing aids to maintain their optimal functioning in the school setting. In a similar manner, some highly externalizing children will need ongoing behavioral support to maintain their own optimal functioning, and supportive services professionals should advocate for the child's right to that support.

APPENDIX A. ANGER COPING PROGRAM
TEACHER NOMINATION

To the Teacher:

Please think about the pupils in your classroom and identify those children who seem to fit *at least three of the five statements* below to some degree. Please feel free to be "liberal" in your selection; we will narrow it down later.

1. The child has marked difficulties with interpersonal problem solving; seems to argue or fight with other children more than most.
2. The child is prone to anger management problems and may use both physical and nonphysical aggression against peers at rates higher than most.
3. The child is frequently disruptive and gives oppositional responses to teacher directives.
4. The child seems to be rejected by the more adaptive children in the class.
5. The child is having academic failure or underachievement problems.

Please list the names below. Rank ordering or filling in all of the slots is not necessary.

_____   _____

_____   _____

_____   _____

_____   _____

_____   _____

Teacher name:_____ Room: _____

APPENDIX B. ANGER COPING PROGRAM
TEACHER SCREENING SCALE

Child's Name _____ School _____ Teacher _____

1. When teased, fights back*   1: Never   2   3   4   5: Almost always

2. Blames others in fights*   1: Never   2   3   4   5: Almost always

3. Overreacts angrily to accidents*   1: Never   2   3   4   5: Almost always

4. Teases and name calls   1: Never   2   3   4   5: Almost always

5. Starts fights with peers   1: Never   2   3   4   5: Almost always

6. Gets into verbal arguments   1: Never   2   3   4   5: Almost always

7. When frustrated, quick to fight   1: Never   2   3   4   5: Almost always

8. Breaks rules in games   1: Never   2   3   4   5: Almost always

9. Responds negatively when fails   1: Never   2   3   4   5: Almost always

10. Uses physical force to dominate**   1: Never   2   3   4   5: Almost always

11. Gets others to gang up on a peer**   1: Never   2   3   4   5: Almost always

12. Threatens and bullies others**   1: Never   2   3   4   5: Almost always

Global Rating _____
Reactive Aggression Rating (sum of items 1, 2, and 3): _____

*Reactive aggressive; **proactive aggressive.

_____

APPENDIX C. ANGER COPING
CLASSROOM GENERALIZATION IN-SERVICE GUIDE

Session 1

Get acquainted; learn the rules about points and strikes; come up with other behavioral expectations; begin learning about individual differences.

In the Classroom: Does the child know the time and date of next meeting? Does he or she know why he or she is in the Anger Coping group? Does he or she know the rules? Does he or she enter and leave the classroom appropriately when group time arrives?

Session 2

Goal setting is explained and initial classroom behavioral goals are written. (Note: The child will have a new Goal Sheet each week for the duration of the group.)

In the Classroom: Does the child spontaneously explain his or her goal to you? Does he or she demonstrate an effort to achieve this goal? Does he or she ask for your initials on his or her Goal Sheet regularly and at the appropriate time? Does he or she reference his or her goal in casual conversation with you? Is his or her goal too difficult to achieve at this time? Can it be modified to be more effective?

Session 3

Begin training in the use of self-instruction—talking silently to yourself—to maintain anger control; puppet self-control exercise is used for the first time.

In the Classroom: Watch for possible excitement carried over from the group. Does the child understand the purpose of the puppet self-control exercise? Watch for the child bragging about his or her puppet's verbal taunting and help him or her turn it around to describing the puppet's self-control instead. Does the child demonstrate an incident of anger control and, spontaneously or when queried, attribute it to self-talk? Reinforce any effort at anger control, including walking away or seeking an adult.

Session 4

Continue training in the use of self-instruction for anger control using direct verbal taunts.

In the Classroom: Watch for possible excitement carried over from the group. Does the child understand the purpose of the taunting exercise? Watch for the child bragging about his or her verbal taunting and help him or her turn it around to describing his or her own self-control instead. What did he or she say to him- or herself to keep from getting angry? Would those words work in the classroom or at recess? Does the child demonstrate an incident of anger control and, spontaneously or when queried, attribute it to self-talk? Reinforce any effort at anger control. Remind the child, "Use your self-talk!" Model your own self-talk where and when appropriate.

Session 5

Begin training in understanding concepts of empathy and perspective taking—for example, "Can you see why that might be fun for you but not for him (or her)?" Begin understanding problem recognition as a difference in perspective or understanding a situation from another's viewpoint.

In the Classroom: Encourage opportunities for problem recognition during conflict situations—for example, "Charles, how do you see the problem? Now, Jason, how do you see the problem?" Model individual perspective taking aloud where and when appropriate— that is, your perspective versus the child's.

Session 6

Continue training in problem recognition; assist the children to understand the feeling of anger—the feeling they have when they think they cannot get something they want, or do something they want to do, or when they feel provoked.

In the Classroom: Continue encouragement of problem recognition. Help the child to label his or her own feelings—for example, "You seem angry (or sad, or frightened, or happy). Tell me why." Or, "Tell me what you're feeling now." As always, reinforce evidence of anger control when observed.

Session 7

Training in the physiological cues to anger—how the child's body feels when he or she is getting angry; begin training in the mediating role of thoughts in anger management—how what you say to yourself can get you more angry or less angry.

In the Classroom: Assist the child in recognizing his or her own anger cues by asking the child to describe them; model aloud your own anger cues in an authentic situation—for example, "I know I'm starting to get angry because I feel my heart starting to pound, so I want you two to get to work."

Session 8

Training in generating alternative responses to problem situations and evaluating possible consequences.

In the Classroom: Ask for alternative responses to authentic problem situations—for example, "What else could you have done? And what else?" Help the child anticipate possible consequences in his or her response selection—for example, "What would probably happen if you did that?" This is also an excellent exercise for the class as a whole.

Session 9

Training in following a sequential problem-solving model: (1) What is the problem? (2) What are my feelings? (3) What are my choices? (4) What will happen if? (5) What will I do?

In the Classroom: Continue to assist the child's efforts to address ambiguous or conflict situations as problems to be addressed. When possible and safe, put the responsibility for nonaggressive conflict resolution with the child—for example, "Jared, I can see you're angry with William. Can you solve this problem so that it turns out best for both of you?" Consider teaching the process to the class as a whole.

Session 10

Continued training in the problem-solving model.

In the Classroom: Continue as in previous session. The teacher should begin to communicate to the child higher expectations for anger management and problem resolution. Continued verbal praise for effective efforts and open notice of his or her changes for the better as they may be demonstrated.

Session 11

Starting at about this session, the group will be making their own videotape in which they will demonstrate what they have learned in the way of anger control and problem solving.

In the Classroom: Inquire as to the progress of the video. What scenarios have been chosen to be taped? How are things going? What skills are you practicing for the video? The teacher should continue to communicate to the child higher expectations for anger management and problem resolution. Continued verbal praise for effective efforts and open notice of the child's changes for the better as they may be demonstrated.

APPENDIX D. MY GOAL SHEET

Name _____   Goal Sheet Number _____

Today's date _____

A goal is something I want to get or something I want to have happen, and I am willing to work for it.

My goal is:

for at least _____ out of five days.

Group member's signature _____

Group leader's signature _____

My teacher will write "Yes" and initial if I met my goal for the day, or "No" and initial if I did not.

	Day 1	Day 2	Day 3	Day 4	Day 5
Teacher initials	_____	_____	_____	_____	_____

Weekly goal met? (circle)   Yes!!   Not yet   Date _____

Name _____

Target goal:_____

_____

Possible behaviors (see Chapter 3)

+1 _____   −1 _____

+2 _____   −2 _____

Great!	Improving	Same	Worse	Poorly
+2	+1	0	−1	−2

Date _____   Teacher initials _____

Great!	Improving	Same	Worse	Poorly
+2	+1	0	−1	−2

Date _____   Teacher initials _____

Great!	Improving	Same	Worse	Poorly
+2	+1	0	−1	−2

Date _____   Teacher initials _____

Great!	Improving	Same	Worse	Poorly
+2	+1	0	−1	−2

Date _____   Teacher initials _____

Great!	Improving	Same	Worse	Poorly
+2	+1	0	−1	−2

Date _____   Teacher initials _____

APPENDIX F. SAMPLE PARENTAL CONSENT LETTER

(Use school letterhead and send over Principal's or Administrator's signature.)

Dear Parent/Guardian:

Your child, _____, is being asked to take part in a small counseling group. The group is called Anger Coping. Your child is being asked to take part in this group because the teacher and I believe that it will help in reaching one or more of these goals we have for the group:

1. Help the children improve control of their anger or tempers
2. Help the children improve their behavior in school
3. Help the children improve their problem-solving skills and set positive classroom goals

The group will meet here at school for about_____ weeks. We will meet on (day or days). The group leader in charge will be _____. He/she can be reached at (phone number).

There are no foreseeable risks that come with participation in this group. Every effort will be made to see that your child misses as little classroom instruction as possible. The teacher will see to it that your child will have makeup time, if needed.

In the group, the children will use role playing to learn anger control skills, how to solve problems with other students or adults, and how to set and meet classroom goals. This is a skills group related primarily to self-control in school. Non-school-related issues are not typically addressed. A full explanation of each activity is available by calling the group leader at the number above. Please call if you have questions or to arrange a meeting here at school. Your support is very important. If, however, you decide that you do not want your child to participate, please know that we will continue to work with him or her in the classroom to be the best student possible. Similar services may be available in the community. Please call for this information if you are interested.

You, your child, and/or the teacher may be asked to complete a checklist so that the group leader can better help your child in the group. The results will be kept confidential, though as the parent or guardian, you are free to inspect them or obtain a copy if you desire. The checklists that will be used are:

_____   _____

Please sign and return the tear-off below. Keep the top for your files.

Sincerely,

_____

(Principal/Administrator)

- -

(Check one)

_____ I give my permission for my child, _____, to take part in the Anger Coping group described above.

_____ I do NOT give my permission.

_____   _____
           Signature   Date

APPENDIX G. ANGER COPING CHECKLIST

Group starting date _____ Times _____

____ Parental consents obtained and filed
____ Co-leader identified
____ Pregroup assessments complete
____ Room secured
____ VCR/monitor reserved
____ Camcorder reserved
____ Teacher(s) consulted on individual classroom goals for Goal
      Setting in Session 2
____ Behavior management strategies designed
____ Reinforcers identified and obtained, if needed
____ DUSO or *Second Step* card obtained for Sessions 1 and 5
____ Hand puppets obtained for Session 3
____ Dominoes and deck of cards obtained for Session 4
____ Transition rules and behavior explained and practiced

Group members:

1. _____   Grade: ____   Room: ____

2. _____   Grade: ____   Room: ____

3. _____   Grade: ____   Room: ____

4. _____   Grade: ____   Room: ____

5. _____   Grade: ____   Room: ____

6. _____   Grade: ____   Room: ____

7. _____   Grade: ____   Room: ____

NOTES:

APPENDIX H. HASSLE LOG

Name _____ Date _____

WHERE WAS I?

____ In my classroom   ____ In the gym

____ In the hall   ____ In the lunchroom

____ On the playground   ____ _____

WHAT HAPPENED?

____ Someone hit or pushed me ____ Someone teased me

____ Someone took something   ____ Someone told me to do
     of mine   something

____ Someone said, "No"   ____ _____

WHAT DID I DO?

____ Used Anger Coping   ____ Hit or pushed the person

____ Yelled and screamed   ____ Walked away, left

____ Sulked or pouted   ____ Told an adult

HOW ANGRY WAS I? (Circle)

Furious!   Pretty Angry   Irritated   Annoyed, but okay

10 9 8   7 6 5   4 3   2 1

HOW DID I HANDLE MYSELF?

____ Great! I really controlled my anger.

____ Pretty well. I tried to use what I have learned.

____ Not so well. I still had trouble with my anger.

APPENDIX I. ANGER COPING PARENT LETTERS

Parent Letter 1

Dear Parents:

Thank you for allowing your child to participate in the Anger Coping group. We are off to a very good start and look forward to helping the children to learn many new skills. Once again, we will be meeting on _____. The members of the group have begun working on personal goals that will help them improve their schoolwork and behavior in the classroom. The group members came up with their own personal goals. Our group session always starts by reviewing these goals and encouraging the children to work hard to meet them.

Most of the goals have to do with getting along with others in school, improving class work, or listening to and obeying the teacher. Once the children have met their goals, they will begin work on new ones.

HOW YOU CAN HELP

♦ Ask your child to discuss his or her goal with you. Why was it important? What are the plans for meeting this goal?
♦ How will your child know when the goal has been met? What problems might be encountered? What are the plans for dealing with those problems?

If three or four times a week you say, "Tell me how you are doing on your Anger Coping goal," your child will understand that what is important at school is also important at home. You may also want to have your child start to set goals for behavior around the home too.

Yours sincerely,

_____

- -

Use this tear-off only if you want to send back any comments or questions you have about the Anger Coping group. Be sure to leave a phone number and "best times to call" if you want me to phone you about your concern.

Your name: _____

Parent Letter 2

Dear Parents:

We are well under way in our Anger Coping group. Recently, we have been working on ways to control the feeling of anger. Lots of children have trouble keeping their tempers under control. In our group, we have been practicing some methods for "keeping your cool." The group members are learning that *what they think or say to themselves* as they start to become angry is very important.

For instance, in our group we have worked on an activity in which the group members actually try to make one another angry. But instead of getting really upset, the children are learning to stay in control by paying attention to what they say to themselves.

HOW YOU CAN HELP

♦ Ask your child to discuss "The Puppet Self-Control" activity. What did the puppet in the circle do to keep from getting too angry?
♦ Ask your child to discuss what he or she did when he or she was in the "safety circle" without the puppet and the others tried to make your child angry. What did your child do to keep from losing his or her temper?
♦ Discuss with your child what you do when you want to "keep your cool" and how important that skill is for you.

Controlling anger is important at home too. Reminding your child to "use your Anger Coping" will help when problems come up at home.

Yours sincerely,

_____

- -

Use this tear-off only if you want to send back any comments or questions you have about the Anger Coping group. Be sure to leave a phone number and "best times to call" if you want me to phone you about your concern.

Your name: _____

Parent Letter 3

Dear Parents:

We have begun to work on one of the most important skills in Anger Coping: How to solve problems with other people. This can include problems with other kids, teachers or other grown-ups, and, of course, problems with parents. To do this, the children have been learning to approach problems by asking a series of "problem-solving questions." The questions are these:

What is the problem? (Stated as *the child's* problem, not the other person's)
What are my feelings? (Is what I feel anger? Am I afraid? Am I sad?)
What are my choices? (Problems often have a number of solutions, good and bad)
What will happen? (Each solution will have consequences)

HOW YOU CAN HELP

- Ask your child to discuss his or her understanding of the problem-solving questions. Do they make sense? Are they helpful?
- See if your child can apply the questions to a problem that may be occurring at home. Was that helpful in reaching a satisfactory solution?

If your children see and hear *you* using the questions to solve a problem of your own, it may help them to learn the skill themselves. I often use this "thinking out loud" method in the group. Try it. You may like it!! Call me if you would like some help with this.

Yours sincerely,

_____

- -

Use this tear-off only if you want to send back any comments or questions you have about the Anger Coping group. Be sure to leave a phone number and "best times to call" if you want me to phone you about your concern.

Your name: _____

APPENDIX J. SAMPLE PARENT CONSENT LETTER AND ANGER COPING PARENT LETTERS SPANISH VERSIONS

Estimados Padres:

Su hijo ha sido seleccionado para tomar parte en un pequeño grupo de terapía. El grupo se llama "Anger Coping" (Canalizar Enojos). Su hijo ha sido seleccionado para tomar parte de este grupo porque su maestro(a) y yo consideramos que esto le ayudará en uno o más de estos objetivos o metas:

1. Ayudará al niño a controlar mejor sus enojos y reacciones negativas.
2. Ayudará al niño a mejorar su conducta en la escuela.
3. Ayudará al niño a mejorar sus abilidades para resolver/solucionar conflictos y a seleccionar metas positivas en el salón de clases.

El grupo se reunirá en la escuela aproximadamente por _____ semanas, todos los _____. El encargado del grupo será _____, a quien usted podrá contactar llamando al _____. Se hará todo el esfuerzo posible para que el niño no pierda mucho tiempo de clase y su maestro(a) le dará tiempo adicional para terminar los trabajos, si fuera necesario.

En el grupo, los niños intractuarán para aprender cómo controlar sus enojos, cómo resolver conflictos con otros niños y adultos, y también trabajarán en el salón de clases para lograr las metas fijadas. Este es un grupo diseñado para enseñar primordialmente cómo obtener control sobre uno mismo en la escuela. Ningún tópico que no sea relacionado con la escuela será discutido en el grupo. Una explicación completa de cada actividad estará a su disposición con sólo llamar al número de teléfono antes mencionado. Por favor llame si tiene alguna pregunta o si desea hacer una cita en la escuela. Su cooperación es muy importante, si por alguna razón usted decidiera que su niño no participe en el grupo, nosotros seguiremos trabajando con él en el salón de clases para que pueda ser un buen estudiante. Servicios similares a éste pueden encontrarse en la comunidad. Siéntase en la libertad de llamar si desea más información o si esta interesado(a).

Usted, su hijo y/o el maestro de su hijo pueden ser contactados para completar un formulario para que el encargado del grupo pueda ayudar mejor a su hijo. Los resultados de éstos formularios seran guardados confidencialmente, aunque ustedes cómo padres tienen la libertad de verlos si desean. Los formularios que se utilizaran son:

_____   _____

Por favor firme y devuelva el talonario que se encuentra al final de ésta carta. Conserve la parte de arriba de ésta carta para su información.

Sinceramente,

_____
(Principal/Administrador)

- -

(Escoja uno)

_____ Yo autorizo a mi hijo, _____, para participar en el grupo "Anger Coping" (Canalizar Enojos), descrito arriba.

_____ Yo NO autorizo.

_____   _____
          Firma   Fecha

Carta a los Padres 1

Estimados Padres:

Gracias por permitirle a su hijo participar en el grupo "Anger Coping" (Canalizar Enojos). Hemos tenido un buen comienzo y esperamos ayudar a que su hijo aprenda nuevas habilidades. Una vez más, nos estamos reuniendo los _____ a las _____.

Los miembros del grupo han comenzado a trabajar en las metas personales que los ayudarán a mejorar sus trabajos escolares y su conducta en el salón de clases. Cada miembro del grupo fijó su propia meta. Nuestras reuniones siempre comienzan repasando esas metas y animando a que los niños trabajen duro para lograrlas.

La mayoría de las metas estan relacionadas a cómo llevarse bien con otros niños en la escuela, como mejorar el trabajo de la clase ó escuela, y a major escuchar y obedecer al maestro (a). Una vez que el niño haya realizado su meta, éste comenzara con una nueva meta.

COMO USTED PUEDE AYUDAR:

♦ Pídale a su hijo que le cuente/platique sus metas a usted. ¿Porqué desidió que era importante? ¿Cuáles son sus planes para realizar esa metas?

♦ ¿Cómo sabrá él cuándo ha realizado su meta? ¿Qué problemas podría tener él? ¿Cuáles son sus planes para enfrentarse con esos problemas?

Si de tres o cuatro veces por semana usted dice, "Dime, cómo te va con la meta de 'Anger Coping' (Canalizar Enojos)," él entenderá que lo que es importante en la escuela también es importante en casa.

Sinceramente,

_____

- -

Use la parte de abajo sólo si usted quiere enviar cualquier comentario o pregunta sobre el grupo. Este seguro de dejar su número de teléfono y "la mejor hora para hablarle" si usted quiere que le llame con relacion a su comentario. Favor de regresar la forma son su hijo al maestro.

Su nombre: _____

Carta a los Padres 2

Estimados Padres:

Vamos bien en nuestro grupo de Anger Coping. Recientemente hemos estado trabajando en diversos metodos para controlar nuestros sentimientos de coraje. Muchos niños tienen problemas manteniendo su temperamento bajo control. En nuestro grupo, hemos estado practicando algunos metodos para "como mantenerse calmado." Los miembros del grupo estan aprendiendo que lo que ellos piensan y se dicen asi mismos cuando se enojan es bien importante.

Por ejemplo, en nuestro grupo hemos estado trabajando en una actividad en la cual los miembros del grupo intentan hacerce enoja unos a otros. Pero, en vez de enojarse los niño estan aprendiendo a mantenerse en control, poniendo atención a lo que se dicen asi mismos.

COMO USTED PUEDE AYUDAR:

♦ Pregunte a su hijo sobre la actividad "El auto-control de la Marioneta." ¿Qué hicieron las marionetas en el circulo pare evitar enojarse?
♦ Pregunte a su hijo lo que hizo cuando estaba dentro del "circulo de seguridad" sin su marionata y los demas niños trataban de hacerle enojar. ¿Qué hizo para no perder el control?
♦ Platique con su hijo que hacer cuanto usted quiere "mantenerse en control" y cuan importante es esa abilidad para usted.

Controlar los enojos es algo muy importante en la casa tambien. Recuerde a su hijo de usar las abilidades aprendidas en el grupo de "Anger Coping" (Canalizando Enojos), esto lo ayudara a resolver problemas que tenga en su casa.

Sinceramente,

_____

- -

Use la parte de abajo sólo si usted quiere enviar cualquier comentario o pregunta sobre el grupo. Este seguro de dejar su número de teléfono y ála mejor hora para hablarle" si usted quiere que le llame con relacion a su comentario. Favor de regresar la forma son su hijo al maestro.

Su nombre: _____

Carta a los Padres 3

Estimados Padres:

Hemos comenzado a trabajar en una de las abilidades más importantes en "Anger Coping" (Canalizar Enojos): Cómo solucionar problemas con otras personas. Esto puede incluir problemas con otros niños, maestros u otros adultos, y por supuesto, problemas con los padres. Para lograr ésto, los niños han estado aprendiendo a enfrentar los problemas por medio de una serie de preguntas. Las preguntas son estas:

¿Qué/Cual es el problema? (Exponiendolo como su problema no el de otras personas)
¿Cuales son mis sentimientos? (¿Es enojo?, ¿Estoy asustado?)
¿Cuales son mis opciones? (Los problemas con frequencia tienen varias soluciones, buenas y malas)
¿Qué podra pasar? (Cada solución tiene una consequencia)

Si su niño lo ve y escucha utilizando éstas preguntas para resolver un problema suyo, esto podra a ayudarlo a aprender esta abilidad por si mismo. Yo uso con frequencia este proceso de pensar en voz alta en el grupo. Tratelo. Puede ser que a usted le guste!! Puede llamarme si desea alguna ayuda.

Sinceramente,

_____

- -

Use la parte de abajo sólo si usted quiere enviar cualquier comentario o pregunta sobre el grupo. Este seguro de dejar su número de teléfono y "la mejor hora para hablarle" si usted quiere que le llame con relacion a su comentario. Favor de regresar la forma son su hijo al maestro.

Su nombre: _____

Recommended Further Reading

◆

Coie, J. D., Underwood, M., & Lochman, J. E. (1991). Programmatic intervention with aggressive children in the school setting. In D. J. Pepler & K. H. Rubin (Eds.), *Development and treatment of childhood aggression* (pp. 389–445). Hillsdale, NJ: Erlbaum.

> *Offers a cogent rationale and perspective for the treatment of anger and aggression in the school setting. The edited volume is an essential for the group leader's library.*

Larson, J. D. (1994). Violence prevention in the schools: A review of selected programs and procedures. *School Psychology Review, 23,* 151–164.

Larson, J. D., Smith, D. C., & Furlong, M. J. (2002). Best practices in school violence prevention. In A. Thomas & J. Grimes (Eds.), *Best practices in school psychology IV.* Bethesda, MD: National Association of School Psychologists.

> *Both references help the practitioner place the Anger Coping Program within the context of a multilevel, school-based prevention program.*

Lochman, J. E., Dunn, S. E., & Wagner, E. E. (1997). Anger. In G. Bear, K. Minke, & A. Thomas (Eds.), *Children's needs II* (pp. 149–160). Bethesda, MD: National Association of School Psychologists.

> *A comprehensive discussion of anger as a mental health concern in children and youth, with references to numerous treatment options.*

Lochman, J. E., FitzGerald, D. P., & Whidby, J. M. (1999). Anger management with aggressive children. In C. Schaefer (Ed.), *Short-term psychotherapy groups for children* (pp. 301–349). Northvale, NJ: Jason Aronson.

Lochman, J. E., Lampron, L. B., Gemmer, T. C., & Harris, S. R. (1987). Anger-coping interventions for aggressive children: Guide to implementation in school settings. In P. A. Keller & S. Heyman (Eds.), *Innovations in clinical practice: A source book* (Vol. 6, pp. 339–356). Sarasota, FL: Professional Resource Exchange.

Lochman, J. E., Lampron, L .B., Gemmer, T. C., Harris, S. R., & Wyckoff, G. M. (1989). Teacher consultation and cognitive-behavioral interventions with aggressive boys. *Psychology in the Schools, 26,* 179–188.

Lochman, J. E., Magee, T. N., & Pardini, D. (in press). Cognitive behavioral interventions for aggressive children. In M. Reinecke & D. Clark (Eds.), *Cognitive therapy over the lifespan: Theory, research and practice.* Cambridge, England: Cambridge University Press.

Lochman, J. E., & Szczepanski, R. G. (1999). Externalizing conditions. In V. L. Schwean & D. H. Saklofske (Eds.), *Psychosocial correlates of exceptionality* (pp. 219–246). New York: Plenum.

Lochman, J. E., Whidby, J. M., & FitzGerald, D. P. (2000). Cognitive-behavioral assessment and treatment with aggressive children. In P. C. Kendall (Ed.), *Child and adolescent therapy: Cognitive-behavioral procedures* (2nd ed., pp. 31–87). New York: Guilford Press.

These references offer further insight into both the theoretical foundation and the research base for the interested practitioner or researcher.

Smith, D. C., Larson, J. D., DeBaryshe, B. D., & Salzman, M. (2000). Anger management for youth: What works and for whom? In D. S. Sandhu (Ed.), *Violence in American schools: A practical guide for counselors* (pp. 217–230). Reston, VA: American Counseling Association.

This chapter is a meta-analysis of the effectiveness of the group anger management programs for children and youth currently available in the research literature.

References

♦

Achenbach, T. M. (1991). *Manual for the Child Behavior Checklist/4–18 and 1991 profile.* Burlington, VT: University of Vermont Department of Psychiatry.

Adler, A. (1964). *Social interest: A challenge to mankind.* New York: Capricorn.

American Guidance Service. (2001). *Developing understanding of self and others (DUSO).* Circle Pines, MN: Author.

American Psychiatric Association. (1994). *Diagnostic and statistical manual of mental disorders* (4th ed.). Washington, DC: Author.

Asarnow, J. R., & Callan, J. W. (1985). Boys with peer adjustment problems: Social cognitive processes. *Journal of Consulting and Clinical Psychology, 53,* 80–87.

Asher, S. R., & Renshaw, P. D. (1981). Children without friends: Social knowledge and social skills training. In S. R. Asher & J. M. Gottman (Eds.), *The development of children's friendships* (pp. 273–296). New York: Cambridge University Press.

Attar, B., Guerra, N., & Tolan, P. (1994). Neighborhood disadvantage, stressful life events, and adjustment in urban elementary school children. *Journal of Clinical Child Psychology, 23,* 391–400.

Bandura, A. (1971). *Social learning theory.* New York: General Learning Press.

Bandura, A. (1973). *Aggression: A social learning analysis.* Englewood Cliffs, NJ: Prentice-Hall.

Bandura, A. (1983). Psychological mechanisms of aggression. In R. G. Geen & E. I. Donnerstein (Eds.), *Aggression: Theoretical and empirical reviews* (Vol. 1, pp. 1–40). San Diego, CA: Academic Press.

Bandura, A., & Barb, P. (1973). Processes governing disinhibatory effects through symbolic modeling. *Journal of Abnormal Psychology, 82,* 1–9.

Bandura, A., & Walters, R. H. (1959). *Adolescent aggression.* New York: Ronald Press.

Barkley, R. A. (1997). *Defiant children* (2nd ed.): *A clinician's manual for assessment and parent training.* New York: Guilford Press.

173

Barkley, R. A. (1998). *Attention-deficit hyperactivity disorder: A handbook for diagnosis and treatment* (2nd ed.). New York: Guilford Press.

Batsche, G. M. . (1998). Bullying. In G. G. Bear, K. M. Minke, & A. Thomas (Eds.), *Children's needs II: Development, problems, and alternatives* (pp. 171–179). Bethesda, MD: National Association of School Psychologists.

Bersoff, D. (1975). Professional ethics and legal responsibilities: On the horns of a dilemma. *Journal of School Psychology, 13,* 359–376.

Bloomquist, M. L., August, G. J., Cohen, C., & Doyle, A., et al. (1997). Social problem solving in hyperactive–aggressive children: How and what they think in conditions of automatic and controlled processing. *Journal of Clinical Psychology, 26*(2), 172–180.

Brestan, E. V., & Eyberg, S. M. (1998). Effective psychosocial treatment of conduct-disordered children and adolescents: 29 years, 82 studies, and 5,272 kids. *Journal of Clinical Child Psychology, 27,* 180–189.

Brown, D., Pryzwansky, W. B., & Schulte, A. C. (1995). *Psychological consultation: Introduction to theory and practice* (2nd ed.). New York: Allyn & Bacon.

Busse, R. T., & Beaver, B. R. (2000). Informant report: Parent and teacher interviews. In E. S. Shapiro & T. R. Kratochwill (Eds.), *Conducting school-based assessments of child and adolescent behavior* (pp. 235–273). New York: Guilford Press.

Charlebois, P., LeBlanc, M., Gagnon, C., & Larivee, S. (1994). Methodological issues in multiple-gating screening procedures for antisocial behaviors in elementary students. *Remedial and Special Education, 15,* 44–54.

Coie, J. D., Lochman, J. E., Terry, R., & Hyman, C. (1992). Predicting early adolescent disorder from childhood aggression and peer rejection. *Journal of Consulting and Clinical Psychology, 60,* 783–792.

Coie, J. D., Terry, R., Zakriski, A., & Lochman, J. E. (1995). Early adolescent social influences on delinquent behavior. In J. McCord (Ed.), *Coercion and punishment in long-term perspectives* (pp. 229–244). Cambridge, England: Cambridge University Press.

Coie, J. D., Underwood, M., & Lochman, J. E. (1991). Programmatic intervention with aggressive children in the school setting. In D. J. Pepler & K. H. Rubin (Eds.), *Development and treatment of childhood aggression* (pp. 389–445). Hillsdale, NJ: Erlbaum.

Committee for Children. (2001). *Second step violence prevention curriculum.* Seattle, WA: Author.

Conduct Problems Prevention Research Group. (1992). A developmental and clinical model for the prevention of conduct disorder: The Fast Track Program. *Development and Psychopathology, 4,* 509–527.

Conduct Problems Prevention Research Group. (1999a). Initial impact of the Fast Track prevention trial for conduct problems: I. The high-risk sample. *Journal of Consulting and Clinical Psychology, 67,* 631–647.

Conduct Problems Prevention Research Group. (1999b). Initial impact of the Fast Track prevention trial for conduct problems: II. Classroom effects. *Journal of Consulting and Clinical Psychology, 67,* 648–657.

Conoley, J. C., & Conoley, C. W. (1992). *School consultation: Practice and training* (2nd ed.). New York: Allyn & Bacon.

Craven, S. (1996). *Examination of the role of physiological and emotional arousal in reactive aggressive boys' hostile attributional biases in peer provocation situations.* Unpublished manuscript, Duke University, Durham, NC.

Crick, N. R. (1997). Engagement in gender normative versus non-normative forms of aggression: Links to social-psychological adjustment. *Developmental Psychology, 33,* 610–617.

Crick, N. R., Bigbee, M. A. (1998). Relational and overt forms of peer victimization: A multi-informant approach. *Journal of Consulting and Clinical Psychology, 66,* 337–347.

Crick, N. R., & Dodge, K. A. (1994). A review and reformulation of social information-processing mechanisms in children's social adjustment. *Psychological Bulletin, 115,* 74–101.

Crick, N. R., & Werner, N. E. (1998). Response decision processes in relational and overt aggression. *Child Development, 69,* 1630–1639.

Cummings, E. M., Iannotti, R. V., & Zahn-Waxler, C. (1985). Influence of conflict between adults on the emotions and aggression of young children. *Developmental Psychology, 21,* 495–507.

Deluty, R. H. (1983). Children's evaluation of aggressive, assertive, and submissive responses. *Journal of Consulting and Clinical Psychology 51,* 124–129.

DeRubeis, R. J., Tang, T. Z., & Beck, A. T. (2001). Cognitive therapy. In K. S. Dobson (Ed.), *Handbook of cognitive-behavioral therapies* (2nd ed., pp. 349–392). New York: Guilford Press.

Derzon, J. H. (2001). Antisocial behavior and the prediction of violence: A meta-analysis. *Psychology in the Schools, 38,* 83–106.

Dishion, T. J., & Andrews, D. W. (1995). Preventing escalation in problem behaviors with high-risk young adolescents: Immediate and 1–year outcomes. *Journal of Consulting and Clinical Psychology, 63,* 538–548.

Dodge, K. A. (1980). Social cognition and children's aggressive behavior. *Child Development, 51,* 162–170.

Dodge, K. A. (1986). A social information processing model of social competence in children. In M. Perlmutter (Ed.), *Cognitive perspectives on children's social and behavioral development: The Minnesota symposium on child psychology* (Vol. 18, pp. 77–125). Hillsdale, NJ: Erlbaum.

Dodge, K. A. (1991). The structure and function of reactive and proactive aggression. In D. J. Pepler & K. H. Rubin (Eds.), *Development and treatment of childhood aggression* (pp. 201–218). Hillsdale, NJ: Erlbaum.

Dodge, K. A. (1993a). Social-cognitive mechanisms in the development of conduct disorder and aggression. *Annual Review of Psychology, 44,* 559–584.

Dodge, K. A. (1993b). The future of research on the treatment of conduct disorder. *Development and Psychopathology, 5,* 311–319.

Dodge, K. A., Bates, J. E., & Pettit, G. S. (1990). Mechanisms in the cycle of violence. *Science, 250,* 1678–1683.

Dodge, K. A., & Coie, J. D. (1987). Social information processing factors in reactive and proactive aggression in children's peer groups. *Journal of Personality and Social Psychology, 53,* 1146–1178.

Dodge, K. A., & Frame, C. L. (1982). Social cognitive biases and deficits in aggressive boys. *Child Development, 53,* 620–635.

Dodge, K. A., Lochman, J. E., Harnish, J. D., Bates, J. E., & Pettit, G. S. (1997). Reactive and proactive aggression in school children and psychiatrically impaired chronically assaultive youth. *Journal of Abnormal Psychology, 106,* 37–51.

Dodge, K. A., Murphy, R. R., & Buchsbaum, K. (1984). The assessment of intention-cue detection skills in children: Implications for developmental psychopathology. *Child Development 55,* 163–173.

Dodge, K. A., & Newman, J. P. (1981). Biased decision-making processes in aggressive boys. *Journal of Abnormal Psychology, 90,* 375–379.

Dodge, K. A., Pettit, G. S., McClaskey, C. L., & Brown, M. M. (1986). Social competence in children. *Monographs of the Society for Research in Child Development, 51*(2, Serial No. 213).

Dollard, J., Doob, L. W., Miller, N. E., Mowrer, O. H., & Sears, R. R. (1939). *Frustration and aggression.* New Haven, CT: Yale University Press.

Donnerstein, E. I., Slaby, R. G., & Eron, L. D. (1994). The mass media and youth aggression. In L. D. Eron, J. H. Gentry, & P. Schlegel (Eds.), *Reason to hope: A psychological perspective on violence and youth* (pp. 383–404). Washington, DC: American Psychological Association.

Dunn, S. E., Lochman, J. E., & Colder, C. R. (1997). Social problem-solving skills in boys with conduct and oppositional disorders. *Aggressive Behavior, 23,* 457–469.

Eisenberg, N., Fabes, R. A., Nyman, M., Bernzweig, J., & Pinuelas, A. (1994). The relations of emotionality and regulation to children's anger-related reactions. *Child Development, 65,* 109–128.

Elliott, S. N., & Gresham, F. M. (1991). *Social skills intervention guide: Practical strategies for social skills training.* Circle Pines, MN: American Guidance Service.

Elliott, S. N., Witt, J. C., Galvin, G., & Peterson, R. (1984). Acceptability of behavior interventions: Factors that influence teachers' decisions. *Journal of School Psychology, 22,* 353–360.

Erdley, C. A. (1990). *An analysis of children's attributions and goals in social situations: Implications of children's friendship outcomes.* Unpublished manuscript, University of Illinois, Champaign, IL.

Eron, L. D., Huesmann, L. R., Dubow, E., Romanoff, R., & Yarmel, P. W. (1987). Aggression and its correlates over 22 years. In D. Crowell, E. Evans, & C. O'Donnell (Eds.), *Aggression and violence: Sources of influence, prevention, and control* (pp. 249–262). New York: Plenum Press.

Eron, L. D., & Slaby, R. G. (1994). Introduction. In L. D. Eron, J. H. Gentry, & P. Schlegel (Eds.), *Reason to hope: A psychological perspective on violence and youth* (pp. 1–22). Washington, DC: American Psychological Association.

Feindler, E. L., Adler, N., Brooks, D., & Bhumitra, E. (1993). The development of the Children's Anger Response Checklist (CARC). In L. VanderCreek (Ed.), *Innovations in clinical practice* (Vol. 12, pp. 337–362). Sarasota, FL: Professional Resources Press.

Feindler, E. L., & Scalley, M. (1999). Adolescent anger-management groups for violence reduction. In T. Kratochwill & K. Stoiber (Eds.), *Handbook of group interventions for children and families* (pp. 100–119). New York: Allyn & Bacon.

Feldman, E., & Dodge, K. A. (1987). Social information processing and sociometric status: Sex, age, and situational effects. *Journal of Abnormal Child Psychology 15,* 211–227.

Fiske, S. T., & Taylor, S. E. (1984). *Social cognition.* Reading, MA: Addison-Wesley.

Forehand, R. L., & McMahon, R. J. (1981). *Helping the noncompliant child: A clinician's guide to parent training.* New York: Guilford Press.

Freeman, A., & Leaf, R. C. (1989). Cognitive therapy applied to personality disorders. In A. Freeman, K. M. Simm, L. E. Beutler, & H. Arkowitz (Eds.), *Comprehensive handbook of cognitive therapy* (pp. 403–433). New York: Plenum Press.

Fuchs, L. S. (1995). Defining student goals and outcomes. In A. Thomas & J. Grimes (Eds.), *Best practices in school psychology III* (pp. 539–546). Bethesda, MD: National Association of School Psychologists.

Furlong, M. J., & Smith, D. C. (Eds.). (1994). *Anger, hostility, and aggression: Assessment, prevention, and intervention strategies for youth.* Brandon, VT: Clinical Psychology.

Goetz, E. T., Hall, R. J., & Fetsco, T. G. (1989). Information processing and cognitive assessment I: Background and overview. In J. N. Hughes & R. J. Hall (Eds.), *Cognitive-behavioral psychology in the schools: A comprehensive handbook* (pp. 87–115). New York: Guilford Press.

Goleman, D. (1995). *Emotional intelligence.* New York: Bantam Books.

Gouze, K R. (1987). Attention and social problem solving as correlates of aggression in preschool males. *Journal of Abnormal Child Psychology, 15,* 181–197.

Guerra, N. G., & Slaby, R. G. (1989). Evaluative factors in social problem solving by aggressive boys. *Journal of Abnormal Child Psychology 17,* 277–289.

Higgins, E. T., King, G. A., & Marvin, G. H. (1982). Individual construct accessibility and subjective impressions and recall. *Journal of Personality and Social Psychology, 43,* 35–47.

Hughes, J. N., & Clavell, T. A. (1995). Cognitive-affective approaches: Enhancing competence in aggressive children. In G. Cartledge & J. F. Miburn (Eds.), *Teaching social skills to children and youth: Innovative approaches* (3rd ed., pp. 199–236). Boston: Allyn & Bacon.

Hughes, J. N., & Hall, R. J. (1987). A proposed model for the assessment of children's social competence. *Professional School Psychology, 2,* 247–260.

Hyman, I., Weiler, E., Perone, D., Romano, L., Britton, G., & Shanock, A. (1997). Victims and victimizers: The two faces of school violence. In A. P. Goldstein & J. C. Conoley (Eds.), *School violence intervention: A practical handbook* (pp. 426–459). New York: Guilford Press.

Ingram, R. E., & Kendall, P. C. (1986). Cognitive clinical psychology: Implications of an informational processing perspective. In R. E. Ingram (Ed.), *Information processing approaches to clinical psychology* (pp. 3–21). New York: Academic Press.

Jacob-Timm, S., & Hartshorne, T. (1998). *Ethics and law for school psychologists* (3rd ed.). New York: Allyn & Bacon.

Joffe, R. D., Dobson, K. S., Fine, S., Marriage, K., & Haley, G. (1990). Social problem-solving in depressed, conduct-disordered, and normal adolescents. *Journal of Abnormal Child Psychology 18,* 565–575.

Jones, R. N., Sheridan, S. M., & Binns, W. R. (1993). Schoolwide social skills training: Providing preventative services to students at risk. *School Psychology Quarterly, 8,* 58–80.

Katsurada, E., & Sugawara, A. I. (1998). The relationship between hostile attributional bias and aggressive behavior in preschoolers. *Early Childhood Research Quarterly 13,* 623–636.

Kaufman, P., Chen, X., Choy, S., Ruddy, S. A., Miller, A. K., Fleury, J. K., Chandler, K. A., Rand, M. R., Klaus, P., & Planty, M. G. (2000). *Indicators of school crime and safety, 2000* (NCES 2001–017). Washington, DC: U.S. Departments of Education and Justice.

Kazdin, A. E. (1982). Symptom substitution, generalization and response covariation: Implications for psychotherapy outcome. *Psychological Bulletin, 91,* 349–365.

Kazdin, A. E. (1987a). Treatment of antisocial behavior in children: Current status and future directions. *Psychological Bulletin, 102,* 187–203.

Kazdin, A. E. (1987b). *Conduct disorders in childhood and adolescence* (Vol. 9). Beverly Hills, CA: Sage.

Kazdin, A. E. (1995). Interventions for aggressive and antisocial children. In L. D. Eron, J. H. Gentry, & P. Schlegel (Eds.), *A reason to hope: A psychosocial perspective on violence and youth* (pp. 341–382). Washington, DC: American Psychological Association.

Kazdin, A. E. (1998). Conduct disorder. In R. J. Morris & T. R. Kratochwill (Eds.), *The practice of child therapy* (3rd ed., pp. 199–230). Boston: Allyn & Bacon.

Kazdin, A. E. (2001). *Behavior modification in applied settings* (6th ed.). Belmont, CA: Wadsworth.

Kazdin, A. E., Siegel, T. C., & Bass, D. (1992). Cognitive problem-solving skills training and parent management training in the treatment of antisocial behavior in children. *Journal of Consulting and Clinical Psychology, 60,* 733–747.

Kazdin, A. E., & Weisz, J. R. (1998). Identifying and developing empirically supported child and adolescent treatments. *Journal of Consulting and Clinical Psychology, 66,* 19–36.

Keane, S. P., & Parrish, A. E. (1992). The role of affective information in the determination of intent. *Developmental Psychology, 28,* 159–162.

Kelly, G. A. (1955). *The psychology of personal constructs.* New York: Norton.

Kendall, P. C. (2000). Guiding theory for therapy with children and adolescents. In P. C. Kendall (Ed.), *Child and adolescent therapy: Cognitive-behavioral procedures* (2nd ed., pp. 3–27). New York: Guilford Press.

Kendall, P. C., Ronan, K. R., & Epps, J. (1991). Aggression in children/adolescents: Cognitive-behavioral treatment perspectives. In D. J. Pepler & K. H. Rubin (Eds.), *Development and treatment of childhood aggression* (pp. 341–360). Hillsdale, NJ: Erlbaum.

Kingery, P. M., Coogeshall, M. B., & Alford, A. A. (1998). Violence at school: Recent evidence from four national surveys. *Psychology in the Schools, 35,* 247–258.

Kiresuk, T. J., Smith, A., & Cardillo, J. E. (Eds.). (1994). *Goal attainment scaling: Application, theory, and measurement.* Hillsdale, NJ: NEA.

Kratochwill, T. R., & Bergan, J. R. (1990). *Behavioral consultation in applied settings.* New York: Plenum Press.

Lahey, B. B., Waldman, I. D., & McBurnett, K. (2001). The development of antisocial behavior: An integrative causal model. *Journal of Child Psychology and Psychiatry, 40,* 669–682.

Larson, J. D. (1993). School psychologists' perceptions of physically aggressive student behavior as a referral concern in nonurban districts. *Psychology in the Schools, 30,* 345–350.

Larson, J. D. (1994). Violence prevention in the schools: A review of selected programs and procedures. *School Psychology Review, 23,* 151–164.

Larson, J. D., Lochman, J. E., & McBride, J. A. (1996). *The Anger Coping Video.* Whitewater, WI: Author.

Larson, J. D., & McBride, J. A. (1993). *Parent to parent: A video-augmented training program for the prevention of aggressive behavior in young children.* Whitewater, WI: Author.

Lochman, J. E. (1984). Psychological characteristics and assessment of aggressive adolescents. In: C. R. Keith (Ed.), *The aggressive adolescent: Clinical perspectives* (pp. 17–62). New York: Free Press.

Lochman, J. E. (1985). Effects of different treatment lengths in cognitive-behavioral interventions with aggressive boys. *Child Psychiatry and Human Development, 16,* 45–56.

Lochman, J. E. (1987). Self and peer perceptions and attributional biases of aggressive and non-aggressive boys in dyadic interactions. *Journal of Consulting and Clinical Psychology, 55,* 404–410.

Lochman, J. E. (1990). Modification of childhood aggression. In M. Hersen, R. Eisler, & P. M. Miller (Eds.), *Progress in behavior modification* (Vol. 2., pp. 47–85). Newbury Park, CA: Sage.

Lochman, J. E. (1992). Cognitive-behavioral interventions with aggressive boys: Three-year follow-up and preventive effects. *Journal of Consulting and Clinical Psychology, 60,* 426–432.

Lochman, J. E. (2000a). Parent and family skills training in targeted prevention programs for at-risk youth. *Journal of Primary Prevention, 21,* 253–265.

Lochman, J. E. (2000b). Theory and empiricism in intervention research: A dialectic to be avoided. *Journal of School Psychology, 38,* 359–368.

Lochman, J. E. (2000c). Conduct disorder. In W. E. Craighead & C. B. Nemeroff (Eds.), *The Corsini encyclopedia of psychology and neuroscience* III. New York: Wiley.

Lochman, J. E. (in press). Preventive intervention with precursors to substance abuse. In W. J. Bukoski & Z. Sloboda (Eds.), *Handbook of drug abuse theory, science, and practice.* New York: Plenum Press.

Lochman, J. E., Burch, P. P., Curry, J. F., & Lampron, L. B. (1984). Treatment and generalization effects of cognitive-behavioral and goal setting interventions with aggressive boys. *Journal of Consulting and Clinical Psychology, 52,* 915–916.

Lochman, J. E., Coie, J. D., Underwood, M., & Terry, R. (1993). Effectiveness of a social relations interventions program for aggressive and nonaggressive rejected children. *Journal of Consulting and Clinical Psychology, 61,* 1053–1058.

Lochman, J. E., & Curry, J. F. (1986). Effects of social problem-solving training and self-instruction training with aggressive boys. *Journal of Consulting and Clinical Psychology, 63,* 549–559.

Lochman, J. E., Dane, H. E., Magee, T. N., Ellis, M., Pardini, B. A., & Claton, N. R. (2001). Disruptive behavior disorders: Assessment and intervention. In B. Vance & A. Pumareigal (Eds.), *The clinical assessment of child and youth behavior: Interfacing intervention with assessment* (pp. 231–262). New York: Wiley.

Lochman, J. E., & Dodge, K. A. (1998). Distorted perceptions in dyadic interactions of aggressive and nonaggressive boys: Effects of prior expectations, context, and boys' age. *Development and Psychopathology, 10,* 495–512.

Lochman, J. E., & Dodge, K. A. (1994). Social-cognitive processes of severely violent, moderately aggressive, and nonaggressive boys. *Journal of Consulting and Clinical Psychology, 62,* 366–374.

Lochman, J. E., Dunn, S. E., & Wagner, E. E. (1997). Anger. In G. Bear, K. Minke & A. Thomas (Eds.), *Children's needs II* (pp. 149–160). Washington, DC: National Association of School Psychology.

Lochman, J. E., FitzGerald, D. P., & Whidby, J. M. (1999). Anger management with aggressive children. In C. Schaefer (Ed.), *Short-term psychotherapy groups for children* (pp. 301–349). Northvale, NJ: Jason Aronson.

Lochman, J. E., & Lampron, L. B. (1986). Situational social problem-solving skills and self-esteem of aggressive and nonaggressive boys. *Journal of Abnormal Child Psychology 14,* 605–617.

Lochman, J. E., & Lampron, L. B. (1988). Cognitive behavioral intervention for aggressive boys: Seven month follow-up effects. *Journal of Child and Adolescent Psychotherapy, 5,* 15–23.

Lochman, J. E., Lampron, L. B., Burch, P. R., & Curry, J. E. (1985). Client characteristics associated with behavior change for treated and untreated boys. *Journal of Abnormal Child Psychology 13,* 527–538.

Lochman, J. E., Lampron, L. B., Gemmer, T. C., & Harris, S. R. (1987). Anger coping intervention with aggressive children: A guide to implementation in school settings. In P. A. Keller & S. R. Heyman (Eds.), *Innovations in clinical practice: A source book* (Vol. 6, pp. 339–356). Sarasota, FL: Professional Resources Exchange.

Lochman, J. E., Lampron, L . B., Gemmer, T. C., Harris, S. R., & Wyckoff, G. M. (1989). Teacher consultation and cognitive-behavioral interventions with aggressive boys. *Psychology in the Schools, 26,* 179–188.

Lochman, J. E., Lampron, L. B., & Rabiner, D. L. (1989). Format and salience effects in the social problem-solving of aggressive and nonaggressive boys. *Journal of Clinical Child Psychology 18,* 230–236.

Lochman, J. E., & Lenhart, L. (1995). Cognitive behavioral therapy of aggressive children: Effects of schemas. In H. P. G. van Bilsen, P. C. Kendall, & J. H. Slavenburg (Eds.), *Behavioral approaches for children and adolescents: Challenges for the next century* (pp. 145–166). New York: Plenum Press.

Lochman, J. E., Magee, T. N., & Pardini, D. (in press). Cognitive behavioral interventions for aggressive children. In M. Reinecke & D. Clark (Eds.), *Cognitive therapy over the lifespan: Theory, research and practice.* Cambridge, England: Cambridge University Press.

Lochman, J. E., Meyer, B. L., Rabiner, D. L., & White, K. J. (1991). Parameters influencing social problem-solving of aggressive children. In R. Prinz (Ed.), *Advances in behavioral assessment of child and families* (Vol. 5, pp. 31–63). Greenwich, CT: JAI Press.

Lochman, J. E., Nelson, W. M., & Sims, J. P. (1981). A cognitive behavioral program for use with aggressive children. *Journal of Clinical Child Psychology 13,* 146–148.

Lochman, J. E., Rahmani, C. H., Flagler, S. L., Nyko-Silva, I., Ross, J. J., & Johnson, J. L. (1998). [Untitled]. Unpublished manuscript, University of Alabama, Tuscaloosa, AL.

Lochman, J. E., & Szczepanski, R. G. (1999). Externalizing conditions. In V. L. Schwean & D. H. Saklofske (Eds.), *Psychosocial correlates of exceptionality* (pp. 219–246). New York: Plenum Press.

Lochman, J. E., & Wayland, K. K. (1994). Aggression, social acceptance, and race as predictors of negative adolescent outcomes. *Journal of the Academy of Child and Adolescent Psychiatry, 33,* 1026–1035.

Lochman, J. E., Wayland, K. K., & White, K. K. (1993). Social goals: Relationship to adolescent adjustment and to social problem solving. *Journal of Abnormal Child Psychology, 21,* 135–151.

Lochman, J. E., & Wells, K. C. (1996). A social-cognitive intervention with aggressive children: Prevention effects and contextual implementation issues. In R. D. Peters & R. J. McMahon (Eds.), *Prevention and early intervention: Childhood disorders, substance use and delinquency* (pp. 111–143). Thousand Oaks, CA: Sage.

Lochman, J. E., & Wells, K. C. (1999a, June). *Effects of an indicated intervention with aggressive boys.* Paper presented at the International Society for Research in Child and Adolescent Psychopathology Ninth Scientific Meeting, Barcelona, Spain.

Lochman, J. E., & Wells, K. C. (1999b, October). *Preventive intervention with preadolescent aggressive children and their parents: The Coping Power Program.* Paper presented at the American Academy of Child and Adolescent Psychiatry Annual Meeting, Chicago, IL.

Lochman, J. E., & Wells, K. C. (1999c, April). *Reactive and proactive aggression in children: Associated child, peer, family and community characteristics.* Paper presented at the Biennial Meeting of the Society for Research in Child Development, Albuquerque, NM.

Lochman, J. E., Wells, K. C., & Colder, C. (1999, September). *Influence of social competence, child, parent, and neighborhood variables on patterns of reactive and proactive aggression in children.* Paper presented at the Life History Research Society Annual Conference, Kauai, HI.

Lochman, J. E., Whidby, J. M., & FitzGerald, D. P. (2000). Cognitive-behavioral assessment and treatment with aggressive children. In P. C. Kendall (Ed.), *Child and adolescent therapy: Cognitive-behavioral procedures* (2nd ed., pp. 31–87). New York: Guilford Press.

Lochman, J. E., White, K. J., Curry, J. F., & Rumer, R. (1992). Antisocial behavior. In V. B. Van Hasselt & D. J. Kolko (Eds.), *Inpatient behavior therapy for children and adolescents* (pp. 277–312). New York: Plenum Press.

Lochman, J. E., White, K. J., & Wayland, K. K. (1991). Cognitive-behavioral assessment and treatment with aggressive children. In P. C. Kendall (Ed.), *Child and adolescent therapy: Cognitive-behavioral procedures* (pp. 25–65). New York: Guilford Press.

Loeber, R. (1990). Development and risk factors of juvenile antisocial behavior and delinquency. *Clinical Psychology Review, 10,* 1–41.

Loeber, R., & Dishion, T. J. (1983). Early predictors of male delinquency: A review. *Psychological Bulletin, 94,* 68–99.

Loeber, R., Dishion, T. J., & Patterson, G. R. (1984). Multiple-gating: A multi-stage assessment procedure for identifying youth at risk for delinquency. *Journal of Research in Crime and Delinquency, 21,* 7–32.

Loeber, R., & Schmalling, K. B. (1985). Empirical evidence for overt and co-vert patterns of antisocial conduct problems: A meta-analysis. *Journal of Abnormal Child Psychology, 13, 337–352.*

Marks, E. S. (1995). *Entry strategies for school consultation.* New York: Guilford Press.

Martens, B. K., & Meller, P. J. (1990). The application of behavioral principles to applied settings. In T. B. Gutkin & C. R. Reynolds (Eds.), *The handbook of school psychology* (2nd ed., pp. 612–634). New York: Wiley.

McConaughy, S. H., & Skiba, R. J. (1993). Comorbidity of externalizing and internalizing problems. *School Psychology Review, 22, 421–436.*

McKinnon, C. E., Lamb, M. E., Belsky, J., and Baum, C. (1990). An affective-cognitive model of mother–child aggression. *Development and Psychopathology 2, 1–13.*

McMahon, R. J., & Estes, A. M. (1997). Conduct problems. In E. J. Mash & L. G. Terdal (Eds.), *Behavioral assessment of childhood disorders* (3rd ed., pp. 130–193). New York: Guilford Press.

McMahon, R. J., & Wells, K. C. (1998). Conduct problems. In E. J. Mash & R. A. Barkley (Eds.), *Treatment of childhood disorders* (2nd ed., pp. 111–207). New York: Guilford Press.

Meichenbaum, D., & Biemiller, A. (1998). *Nurturing independent learners: Helping students take charge of their learning.* Cambridge, MA: Brookline Books.

Milich, R., & Dodge, K. A. (1984). Social information processing in child psychiatric populations. *Journal of Abnormal Child Psychology 12, 471–490.*

Miller, G. (1994). Enhancing family-based interventions for managing childhood anger and aggression. In M. J. Furlong & D. C. Smith (Eds.), *Anger, hostility, and aggression: Assessment, prevention, and intervention strategies for youth* (pp. 83–116). Brandon, VT: Clinical Psychology.

Miltenberger, R. G. (1997). *Behavior modification: Principles and procedures.* Pacific Grove, CA: Brooks/Cole.

Minke, K. M., & Bear, G. G. (2000). *Preventing school problems—Promoting school success: Strategies and programs that work.* Bethesda, MD: National Association of School Psychologists.

Mischel, W. (1990). Personality disposition revisited and revised: A view after three decades. In L. Pervin (Ed.), *Handbook of personality: Theory and research* (pp. 111–134). New York: Guilford Press.

National Association of School Psychologists. (1984). *Principles for professional ethics.* Bethesda, MD: Author.

National School Safety Center. (2001). *School-associated violent deaths report.* [On-line]. Available: http:\\www.nsscl.org.

Nelson, W. M., III, & Finch, A. J. (2000). *Children's inventory of anger.* Los Angeles: Western Psychological Services.

Novaco, R. W. (1978). Anger and coping with stress: Cognitive-behavioral intervention. In J. P. Foreyet & D. P. Rathjen (Eds.), *Cognitive behavioral therapy: Research and application* (pp. 135–173). New York: Plenum Press.

Ogles, B. M., Lambert, M. J., & Masters, K. S. (1996). *Assessing outcomes in clinical practice.* Boston: Allyn & Bacon.

Olweus, D. (1993). *Bullying at school: What we know and what we can do.* Cambridge, MA: Blackwell.

Park, R. D., & Slaby, R. G. (1983). The development of aggression. In E. M. Hetherington (Ed.), *Handbook of child psychology: Vol. 4. Socialization, personality, and social development* (pp. 547–641). New York: Wiley.

Patterson, G. R. (1974). Interventions for boys with conduct problems: Multiple settings, treatments, and criteria. *Journal of Consulting and Clinical Psychology, 42,* 471–481.

Patterson, G. R. (1982). *Coercive family process.* Eugene, OR: Castalia.

Patterson, G. R., DeBaryshe, B. D., & Ramsey, E. (1989). A developmental perspective on antisocial behavior. *American Psychologist, 44,* 329–335.

Patterson, G. R., Reid, J. B., & Dishion, T. J. (1992). *Antisocial boys.* Eugene, OR: Castalia.

Patterson, G. R., Reid, J. B., Jones, R. R., & Conger, R. E. (1975). *A social learning approach to family intervention: Families with aggressive children.* (Vol. 1). Eugene, OR: Castalia.

Pepler, D. J., Craig, W. M., & Roberts, W. I. (1998). Observations of aggressive and nonaggressive children on the school playground. *Merrill–Palmer Quarterly 44* (1), 55–76.

Pepler, D. J., King, G., & Byrd, W. (1991). A social-cognitively based social skills training program for aggressive children. In D. J. Pepler & K. H. Rubin (Eds.), *Development and treatment of childhood aggression* (pp. 361–379). Hillsdale, NJ: Erlbaum.

Pepler, D. J., & Sedighdeilami, F. (1998, October). *Aggressive girls in Canada* (Report No. W-98–30E). Applied Research Branch, Strategic Policy, Human Resources Development Canada, Hull, Quebec, Canada. [On-line]. Available: *http://www.hrdc-drhc.gc.ca/stratpol/arb/publications/research/abw-98–30e.shtml.*

Pepler, D. J., & Slaby, R. G. (1994). Theoretical and developmental perspectives on youth and violence. In L. D. Eron, J. H. Gentry, & P. Schlegel (Eds.). *Reason to hope: A psychological perspective on violence and youth* (pp. 27–58). Washington, DC: American Psychological Association.

Perry, D. G., Perry, L. C., & Rasmussen, P. (1986). Cognitive social learning mediators of aggression. *Child Development, 57,* 700–711.

Pettit, G. S. (1997). Aggressive behavior. In G. C. Bear, K. M. Minke, & A. Thomas (Eds.), *Children's needs II: Development, problems, and alternatives* (pp. 135–148). Bethesda, MD: National Association of School Psychologists.

Prinz, R. J., & Miller, G. E. (1994). Family-based treatment for childhood antisocial behavior: Experimental influences on dropout and engagement. *Journal of Consulting and Clinical Psychology, 62,* 645–650.

Rabiner, D. L., Lenhart, L., & Lochman, J. E. (1990). Automatic vs. reflective problem solving in relation to children's sociometric status. *Developmental Psychology 71,* 535–543.

Reid, J. B., & Patterson, G. R. (1991). Early prevention and intervention with conduct problems: A social interactional model for the integration of research and practice. In G. Stoner, M. R. Shinn, & H. M. Walker (Eds.), *Interventions for achievement and behavior problems* (pp. 715–739). Bethesda, MD: National Association of School Psychologists.

Reynolds, C., & Kamphaus, R. W. (1992). *Behavior assessment system for children (BASC).* Circle Pines, MN: American Guidance Services.

Roff, J. D. (1986). Identification of boys at high risk for delinquency. *Psychological Reports, 58,* 615–618.

Rose, L. C., & Gallup, A. M. (2000). The 31st annual Phi Delta Kappa/Gallup poll of the public's attitude toward the public schools. [On-line]. Available: *http://www.pdkintl.org/kappan/kpol9909.htm.*

Rotter, J. B., Chance, J. E., & Phares, E. J. (1972). *Applications of a social learning theory of personality.* New York: Holt, Rinehart & Winston.

Rubin, K. H., Bream, L. A., & Rose-Krasnor, L. (1991). Social problem solving and aggression in childhood. In D. J. Pepler & K. H. Rubin (Eds.), *The development and treatment of childhood aggression* (pp. 219–248). Hillsdale, NJ: Erlbaum.

Sancilio, M., Plumert, J. M., & Hartup, W. W. (1989). Friendship and aggressiveness as determinants of conflict outcomes in middle childhood. *Developmental Psychology 25,* 812–819.

Shure, M. (1996). *I can problem-solve: An interpersonal cognitive problem-solving program.* Champaign, IL: Research Press.

Sinclair, E., Del'Homme, M., & Gonzalez, G. (1993). Systematic screening for preschool behavioral disorders. *Behavioral Disorders, 18,* 177–188.

Skrtic, T. M. (1991). *Behind special education: A critical analysis of professional culture and school organization.* Denver, CO: Love.

Slaby, R. G., & Guerra, N. G. (1988). Cognitive mediators of aggression in adolescent offenders: An assessment. *Developmental Psychology, 24,* 580–588.

Sladeczek, I. E., Elliott, S. N., Kratochwill, T. R., Robertson-Majaanes, S., & Callan-Stoiber, K. (2001). Application of goal attainment scaling to a conjoint behavioral consultation. *Journal of Educational and Psychological Consultation, 12,* 45–48.

Smith, C. A., & Lazarus, R. W. (1990). Emotion and adaptation. In L. Pervin (Ed.), *Handbook of personality: Theory and research* (pp. 609–637). New York: Guilford Press.

Smith, D. C., Larson, J. D., DeBaryshe, B. D., & Salzman, M. (2000). Anger management for youth: What works and for whom? In D. S. Sandhu (Ed.), *Violence in American schools: A practical guide for counselors* (pp. 217–230). Reston, VA: American Counseling Association.

Sprick, R. (1999). *25 minutes to better behavior: A teacher to teacher problem-solving process.* Longmont, CO: Sopris West.

Steinberg, M. E., & Dodge, K. A. (1983). Attributional bias in aggressive adolescent boys and girls. *Journal of Social and Clinical Psychology, 1,* 312–321.

Tangney, J. P., Wagner, P. E., Hansbarger, A., & Gramzow, R. (1991). *The Anger Response Inventory for Children (ARI-C).* Fairfax, VA: George Mason University Press.

Tharinger, D., & Stafford, M. (1996). Best practices in individual counseling of elementary-age students. In A. Thomas & J. Grimes (Eds.), *Best practices in school psychology III* (pp. 893–907). Bethesda, MD: National Association of School Psychologists.

Thelen, M. H., Fry, R. A., Feherenbach, P. A., & Frautschi, N. M. (1979). Therapeutic videotape and film modeling: A review. *Psychological Bulletin, 86,* 701–720.

Waas, G. A. (1988). Social attributional biases of peer-rejected and aggressive children. *Child Development 59*, 969–975.

Waas, G. A., & French, D. C. (1989). Children's social problem solving: Comparison of the open middle interview and children's assertive behavior scale. *Behavioral Assessment 11*, 219–230.

Walker, H. M., Severson, H. H., Stiller, B., Williams, G., Haring, N., Shinn, M., & Todis, B. (1988). Systematic screening of pupils in the elementary age range at risk for behavior disorders: Development and trial testing of a multiple gating model. *Remedial and Special Education, 9*, 8–14.

Webster-Stratton, C. (1989a). *The parents and children series: A comprehensive course divided into four programs.* Eugene, OR: Castalia.

Webster-Stratton, C. (1989b). Systematic comparison of consumer satisfaction of three cost-effective parent training programs for conduct problem children. *Behavior Therapy, 20*, 103–115.

Webster-Stratton, C. (1992). Individually administered videotape parent training: Who benefits? *Cognitive Therapy and Research, 16*, 31–35.

Webster-Stratton, C., & Hammond, M. (1997). Treating children with early-onset conduct problems: A comparison of child and parent training interventions. *Journal of Consulting and Clinical Psychology, 65*, 93–109.

Webster-Stratton, C., Kolpacoff, M., & Hollinsworth, T. (1988). Self-administered videotape therapy for families with conduct-problem children: Comparison with two cost-effective treatments and a control group. *Journal of Consulting and Clinical Psychology, 56*, 458–565.

Weiner, B., & Graham, S. (1999). Attribution in personality psychology. In L. A. Pervin & O. P. John (Eds.), *Handbook of personality: Theory and research* (2nd ed., pp. 605–628). New York: Guilford Press.

Whebby, J. H., Dodge, K. A., Valente, E., Jr., Bierman, K., Coie, J. D., Greenburg, M., & Lochman, J. E. (1993). School behavior of first grade children identified as at-risk for development of conduct problems. *Behavioral Disorders, 19*, 67–78.

Ysseldyke, J., Dawson, P., Lehr, C., Reschly, D., Reynolds, M., & Telzrow, C (1997). *School psychology: A blueprint for training and practice II.* Bethesda, MD: National Association of School Psychologists.

Yung, B. R., & Hammond, W. R. (1998). Breaking the cycle: A culturally sensitive violence prevention program for African-American children and adolescents. In A. Lutzker (Ed.), *Handbook of child abuse research and treatment* (pp. 319–340). New York: Plenum Press.

Zelli, A., Dodge, K. A., Lochman, J. E., Laird, R. D., & the Conduct Problems Prevention Research Group (1999). The distinction between beliefs legitimizing aggression and deviant processing of social cues: Testing measurement validity and the hypothesis that biased processing mediates the effects of beliefs on aggression. *Journal of Personality and Social Psychology, 77*, 150–166.

Index

♦

DATE DUE

	FEB 2 5 2003		